"With depth, storytelling, and experience, Sarah Ezrin draws from the wisdom of yoga philosophy to bring empathy and appreciation to parenting, reminding readers that parenthood is a valuable and important spiritual practice in its own right. I wish I had *The Yoga of Parenting* when I was raising my kids. Fortunately, the benefits of this book extend to parents like me, who are beyond the early, intensive parenting years. I love this book!"

—Britta Bushnell, PhD, author of *Transformed by Birth*

"Parenthood is a wild ride with many different phases. *The Yoga of Parenting* draws from the yogic tradition and teaches us to embrace the enormous responsibility and privilege of parenting with wisdom and humor. Sarah Ezrin gracefully weaves yoga asanas, personal stories, and the philosophical teachings from many different traditions. Staying grounded as a parent can be challenging on any given day and having real world techniques to guide us is truly a gift!"

—Desi Bartlett, MS, CPT, E-RYT, pre- and postnatal yoga expert, author, and mom

"Mom-ing is hard; yoga can help. This optimistic book offers empathy followed by gentle techniques for grounding and connecting, so that your practice can uplift your parenting."

—Lizzie Lasater, yogi, designer, and mom of twins

"*The Yoga of Parenting* is not just for people familiar with yoga; it is accessible, relatable, and transformative for people with a longtime practice and those who never thought yoga was for them. Sarah skillfully weaves in storytelling, wisdom

and reflection to make this a truly practical guide for parents and caregivers on the messy and humbling journey of raising a human. Raising a child can break us or grow our soul. Yoga philosophy can offer a framework for allowing parenting to be the latter while acknowledging our humanity."

—Hala Khouri, MA, SEP, E-RYT,
author of *Peace from Anxiety*

"*The Yoga of Parenting* is a soothing balm for all of us who have the privilege and challenge of caring for children. It's like a long, slow exhale, creating space for reflection in the midst of the chaos. Sarah Ezrin reminds us that parenting is a spiritual journey made up of opposites—of connection and separation, intimacy and boundaries, inhales and exhales. She offers us yoga teachings and practices to balance those opposites and cultivate a meaningful and peaceful family life."

—Jivana Heyman, author of *Accessible Yoga*
and *Yoga Revolution*

"A central question for many parents who practice yoga is this: how to leverage the structure and power of on-the-mat yoga practice within the constantly changing, unpredictable, and hardly structured real life of being a parent? Sarah Erzin responds to this question in a generous, insightful, and practical way in *The Yoga of Parenting*. Clear-sighted and firmly rooted in the everyday reality of parenting, her book reminds the reader that in the realm of parenting, practice does not make 'perfect'—practice makes possible."

—Octavia Raheem, author of *Pause, Rest, Be* and *Gather*

The YOGA of PARENTING

....

Ten Yoga-Based Practices
to Help You Stay Grounded,
Connect with Your Kids
& Be Kind to Yourself

SARAH EZRIN

Foreword by Jennifer Pastiloff

SHAMBHALA

Shambhala Publications, Inc.
2129 13th Street
Boulder, Colorado 80302
www.shambhala.com

Cover art: Cat Grishaver
Cover design: Cat Grishaver
Interior design: Kate Huber-Parker

9 8 7 6 5 4 3 2 1

First Edition
Printed in the United States of America

Shambhala Publications makes every effort
to print on acid-free, recycled paper.
Shambhala Publications is distributed worldwide by
Penguin Random House, Inc., and its subsidiaries.

Library of Congress Cataloging-in-Publication Data
Names: Ezrin, Sarah, author.
Title: The yoga of parenting: ten yoga-based practices to help you stay
grounded, connect with your kids, and be kind to yourself /
Sarah Ezrin; foreword by Jennifer Pastiloff
Description: Boulder, Colorado : Shambhala, [2023] |
Includes bibliographical references.
Identifiers: LCCN 2022041895 | ISBN 9781645471172 (trade paperback)
Subjects: LCSH: Parent and child—Psychological aspects. |
   Parenting—Psychological aspects. | Yoga.
Classification: LCC BF723.P25 E97 2023 | DDC 155.9/24—dc23/
eng/20220914
LC record available at https://lccn.loc.gov/2022041895

To Ben, Jonah, and Jacob,

thank you for making me a mama.

You are my everythings.

CONTENTS

FOREWORD

I felt like a fraud when Sarah asked me to write this foreword. I looked at my yoga mat—who am I kidding, my thirty yoga mats—all rolled up in random corners of my house, all collecting dust, paint (I'd begun to use them as easels), or my son's Legos and toys that he played with one time before forgetting about.

I saw these former lovers of mine (and they were most certainly lovers at one point) and thought, "Jennifer! What in the name of Downward Dog are you doing saying yes to this book about yoga when you haven't practiced since 1976?" Fine, it had only been a year, maybe. But still. The pandemic has altered time, and everything feels like eight hundred years ago. Or yesterday.

I unrolled one of my less filthy mats and sat on it. I didn't do any stretching or twisting or fancy poses. (Not like I ever did. I was always the one whose favorite pose was *Savasana*.) I just sat there and felt my body begin to settle.

My muscle memory began to kick in and I felt—wait for it—at home.

I felt at home.

"Fine," I said aloud to myself (I do this a lot and without an ounce of shame). "Fine, the body knows. My intuition knows. I just need to trust it."

When Sarah asked me to do this task, I was horrified. What could I possibly say about something I'd abandoned? But my body, my gut, my cellular memory of all that yoga had done for me—it knew: I hadn't stopped doing yoga just because I had not been practicing asana.

And it was reading Sarah's *The Yoga of Parenting* that helped me become even clearer on that fact.

Sarah has a gift for teaching. I've known that since I met her fifteen years ago. The way she transforms her own stories and pain and experiences and victories into opportunities for others to see themselves is nothing short of magical. She does this not only with skill but with vulnerability and humor. You can't help but want to listen to what she has to say, and then you inadvertently learn from her and, voilà, you're a better human.

I'm telling you—this happens.

When someone genuinely shares their passion in the way Sarah does, it's inevitable that you are affected. You won't realize at first how her wisdom has entered you and altered your DNA. I've found that all the best teachers silently creep up on me as I'm sitting at breakfast pouring the coffee. "Ah! Look at my behavior! Look at my thoughts. That's from Sarah's teaching."

I delight in this. It doesn't feel like forced learning, or some yoga influencer on Instagram promising you'll be a better mom if you only feed your kid organic homemade cashew milk before offering you a coupon code for a monthly subscription. No, it is from the heart and, I'd argue, from eight hundred million years of wisdom. Why that long? Because Sarah Ezrin is an old soul, and you'll see that as you highlight every page in here.

I don't question when my teachers show up or how they know what they know. I just appreciate it. I eat it up and I say, "thank you."

Sarah and I are opposites in so many ways, and in so many ways we are the same person. This is one of my favorite parts about being human—how this can be possible with another person and yet we can still feel like we've found our soulmate, our greatest teacher, our lover, or our child. We can always learn so much if only we stay open. If only we stay connected.

Which brings me back to yoga. Yoga is connection and connection is my favorite thing on this planet.

This beautiful book, which I plan to gift to everyone and which I carry around everywhere, has reminded me that yoga and parenting are both about divine connection. It reminded me that all we have to do is simply allow for this connection.

This book offers practices and tools that I love and need—for example, the reminder to keep breathing. While this may seem like an obvious thing, it's something that I forget nine times out of ten. That's a conservative estimate. I'm very committed to being transparent, so there you go. It's the truth. It astounds me how often I forget to breathe. I don't think I'm special in that. A lot of us forget to breathe and walk around with our shoulders up inside our ears.

And if we think that is not affecting our parenting, we are delusional.

Yes, I am often delusional.

And yet every day I decide to begin again, read again, begin again, and with this book, roll out my mat again (once I wipe off the Legos and paint). I'm not neat or organized, and I am still a good mom. I'm still a *great* mom. This book reminds me of that fact. Sarah reminds me of that.

I have one tattoo and it says "I got you," so I hope you realize how important it is to me to be gotten by someone—whether it's in real life or through a beautiful book like this. It is everything. We need our people. Our guides. Our true norths. Sometimes they show up in the form of our children, sometimes they show up in the form of our yoga teachers, sometimes they show up in the form of our spouses, sometimes they show up in the form of the person who bags our groceries, and sometimes they show up in the form of a book.

Perhaps the biggest epiphany I had while reading (and actually it was not an epiphany but more of an "Oh yeah, I forgot that!") was when I came across these words: "Putting our needs aside does not make us better parents. The more disconnected we are from ourselves, the more disconnected we are from everyone else. It is impossible to be fully present with someone when you cannot be fully present with yourself. It is impossible to give someone your all if you have nothing to give."

I felt seen.

I wanted to hide.

Instead, I kept reading. I kept looking inward and asking hard questions and getting back on my mat and following along with what the book was saying because, *duh*, it seemed to know some things.

So while yes, this is a book about yoga and parenting, it is also a book about me.

And you.

My eyes were opened, and I could not shut them again. This book did that—and here I was thinking I was simply going to learn some yoga poses and maybe find some ways to help my son put down the video games.

Nope.

This book was a reckoning with myself and by the end, I was parenting in a way that was in alignment with who I truly am. I was more patient. I was saying yes only when I wanted to and no much more often. I was finding and then doing what lit me up. I was paying attention to my body and my breath. I was taking care of my family and myself in a way I had not in years, if ever. Because, as Sarah reminds us, you must be present with yourself first if you want to be present with others.

This book is for all of us, whether you're a seasoned yogi or you've never set foot on a mat (in which case, yay! You will get to begin); whether you're a parent or a nanny, an auntie, a foster parent, or a godparent; even if you, frankly, don't particularly like children (not judging!).

This book will be a journey into you, you ridiculously unique miracle of a human.

And while I can't say whether you've done a million smart things in your life (I have not, but you might have), I know for certain that you did one really smart thing. You picked up this book, which will change your life and your family. It's like you finally stopped touching the hot stove after burning your hand a thousand times. It's like you finally woke up and said, "Okay, enough. I am ready to come back to myself (and also to stop going near the stinking stove, for the love of Warrior Twos.)"

So it begins.

Jennifer Pastiloff

INTRODUCTION

Parenting has nothing to do with perfection. Perfection isn't even the goal, not for us, not for our children. Learning together to live well in an imperfect world, loving each other despite or even because of our imperfections, and growing as humans while we grow our little humans, those are the goals of gentle parenting. So, don't ask yourself at the end of the day if you did everything right. Ask yourself what you learned and how well you loved, then grow from your answer. That is perfect parenting.

—L. R. Knost, *The Gentle Parent*

My toddler threw a water bottle at his one-week-old baby brother.

It wasn't one of those tiny plastic ones you get in the back of an Uber either. It was a stainless steel sixty-four-ounce bottle that was so heavy, I had to put a grip cover around it to help me hold it with my adult hands. Yet, somehow, my two-and-a-half-year-old not only picked it up but he also threw it a substantial distance.

My sister was holding the baby and, thankfully, the bottle didn't make a physical impact, but that didn't lessen my reaction.

"Jonah!" I exploded. "Why did you do that?"

I took him into his room with a bit more force than I would like to admit and he quickly went from laughing to crying.

I was shaking with anger and tempted to throw something myself, but just as I was about to yell again, I instead chose to take a breath and hugged him toward me.

He started clawing out of my arms, demanding to go back to the living room to keep playing, but as I continued to breathe deeply and my heart rate and anger lessened, I noticed his whole being start to soften too, and suddenly "I want to play" morphed into "I want my mama" and him collapsing into my arms.

He was no monster, despite my nervous system trying to convince me otherwise. He was a little boy whose entire world had just been blown apart with the arrival of the new baby.

His role as our one and only had ended, and no matter how well we tried to prepare him and excite him about his new role as big brother, he was feeling deep grief.

Sure, it appeared on the surface that he was trying to hurt his brother (and maybe there was some intention of that), but when I looked into his big brown eyes with tears beading at the lash line, I knew in my heart he wasn't being malicious. And I was no longer mad.

Taking that single breath afforded me the space to change the trajectory of our family's entire day. Once he was regulated and making eye contact again, I asked him if he wanted to breathe with me. Looking into one another's eyes, we inhaled and exhaled in unison for a few rounds.

After that, I brought him back to the living room with the rest of the family. He got excited again pretty quickly, throwing balls a little too close to his baby brother, but while prior to our "time in" his every move had me on edge, I was now able to laugh and take in the whole scene of the beautiful chaos that is young family life.

YOGA IS CONNECTION

I can say without a shadow of a doubt that were it not for my dedicated daily yoga practice, things would have gone very differently that afternoon. In fact, I can identify many moments in my parenting journey just today that would have had different outcomes were it not for my yoga practice, and I'm not talking about handstands or Warrior Poses either.

The root of yoga is really about connection (the root word, *yuj*, means "to connect"). This means that anything we do with a focused mind and a whole heart is yoga. Gazing at our babies while they suckle, breathing with our toddlers during a tantrum, laughing with our littles while chasing them in the backyard, listening intently to our teenagers as they tell us a story, being present for the entire wild ride that is parenting—this is all yoga.

One of my main goals of writing this book is to encourage us to slow down before reacting within parenthood. Our children are going to do things that test us. They will act out and push limits and have opposing agendas. When we are not grounded or present, we risk operating from reaction mode instead of getting clear on what everyone really needs—which more often than not is some kind of pause or connection.

Having grown up in a household that was wrought with addiction, alcoholism, and explosive anger, I can tell you firsthand that getting present and connecting can prevent explosions that lead to days (or even years) of reparations. Simply taking a breath allows us the space to choose more compassionate and well-thought-out responses.

And this is exactly what we are going to practice together throughout this book. Through the practice of yoga, we will learn how to observe disequilibrium rather than automatically being knocked over by it.

By bringing the wisdom of yoga into your parenting journey, you will gain more presence, patience, and acceptance—with your child and even (and especially) with yourself.

PARENTING IS YOGA

I have been meditating for nearly thirty years and practicing asana, the physical practice, for over twenty and I can say without a doubt that the most advanced yoga I have ever done is raising children.

I have never been more stretched, more challenged, or more strengthened nor have I felt more ecstasy or been more connected than I have raising my two sons. And I used to wrap my legs behind my head every morning before coffee!

When we think of yoga, we often picture someone doing a fancy pose on a beach, but the physical practice is just a tiny piece of this incredible tradition. Yoga is much more about how we live our lives than what shapes we make with our bodies. It is about unity and connection—and who do we want to be more connected to than our children? (Well, most days anyway.)

I have witnessed firsthand how this ancient practice changes how people interact with and behave in the world. I have seen how much kinder, more compassionate, calm, and balanced parents who practice yoga can be.

And I have also seen how incredibly human yoga-practitioner parents still are too; no matter how many spiritual texts we read or hours we sit for meditation, or how many silent retreats we go on, we still yell at our kids. We still cry when we are overwhelmed, and we still need help sometimes (okay, a lot of the time). I mean, even the Dalai Lama admits to getting angry, and he doesn't have children.

The truth is we are all works in progress: "Perfectly imperfect," as the saying goes. And parenting has been and always will be the most challenging personal work some of us will ever do.

Maybe that is why so many spiritual paths encourage renunciation. It is much harder to reach a realized state when your three-year-old is destroying your house and your newborn is scream-crying in the other room.

But this is also why parenthood can be the ultimate spiritual experience. It is no coincidence that I wrote this book while learning to navigate the dynamic of raising both a toddler and a baby. We have an opportunity to learn way more about ourselves when we interact with the world than sitting quietly in a meditative state. As Hunter Clarke-Fields, the author of *Raising Good Humans: A Mindful Guide to Breaking the Reactive Cycle of Parenting and Raising Kind, Confident Kids*, says, "Six months with a preschooler can be more effective than years alone on a mountain top." Adding, "It might just be the fast track to enlightenment."

If we are willing to slow down and look at our stuff, parenthood can provide a powerful lens for us to get to know ourselves more deeply. Much like when we are on our yoga mats, it is a place in our lives where we can observe our tendencies and learn how to shift our behaviors.

As such, this book will be part yoga mat, part mirror, part best friend, part tissue box, and a whole lot of safe space for you to learn how to be more compassionate with your children and yourself.

HEALING POWER OF CONNECTION
AND ACCEPTING OUR IMPERFECTIONS

I found a peace in yoga that is only possible when you are fully and completely present in the moment. It is a contentment only available when deeply in tune to everything and everyone. It is the healing power of connection.

And this experience is not some mythical land or advanced meditation technique that only a few realized beings have mastered. I felt this at twelve years old while learning to meditate on my therapist's couch and when I taught yoga to over one hundred bodies at once. I felt it when I kissed my husband on our wedding day and even just the other day while napping with the baby.

I feel it any time that I am grounded in the moment and fully present with whatever it is that I am doing. This place of connection is available to all of us any time we choose to slow down and become aware. You have already made that choice by simply picking up this book.

As a longtime practitioner and teacher, I have had the privilege to witness the practice of yoga help thousands upon thousands of people be kinder to themselves, more aware of their choices and actions, and more present. I've also witnessed the practice help many people to accept and embrace the fact that we as humans are constantly evolving.

The teachings of yoga remind us of our continual growth, and they teach us that while we are each works in progress, in every phase of that growth, we are still whole. For example, there is a saying that the acorn is perfect in its form, just as the sapling is, and finally, the oak tree.

Similarly, we would never say that our infant is not a whole person, yet we don't expect them to be able to walk and talk right out of the womb. We recognize that they have a lot of growth to do before they get there. So, why do we feel, the minute we bring a child home, that we should know it all?

I wrote this book so that we may learn to give ourselves the same permission to be in progress as we do our children. I wrote it as protection against the external pressures and messages from society telling us we are not doing enough.

Most importantly, I wrote this book to remind us that we and our children are perfect exactly as we are, even and especially because of our imperfections.

EVERYTHING YOU NEED TO KNOW, YOU KNOW

In addition to coming to the mat almost every day for the past twenty years and attending therapy since I was eight years old, I have read a lot of personal development books. Like, a lot.

I find them comforting. Perhaps it's the illusion of taking control when everything feels so out of control? And while I always gain insight, I notice that a lot of the books, especially those in the parenting sector, seem to either offer one-size-fits-all solutions or make you feel as though you must precisely follow that author's plan.

If I have learned anything from my yoga practice and teaching career, it is that these one-size-fits-all approaches do not work on the mat, so why would we expect them to work off the mat?

And why would we expect this to work with our children? People's day-to-days can look completely different with different children in the exact same household (!), let alone from home to home.

We are not cookie-cutter molds of one another. We each come to the table with rich histories and unique present circumstances. Acknowledging these differences helps us see that there is no one right way. There is no perfect.

It also means that the greatest teachers are your children and *you*. Your intuition knows way more than any book or expert or in-law or social media troll.

Now, before you wonder why you are even bothering reading this if I don't plan to tell you what to do, may I offer something? Multiple senior teachers I interviewed for this book—from Matthew Sanford in Minneapolis to Darren Main in the Bay Area—prefer to say that they "share" the practice of yoga with students as opposed to "teaching" it. This is much like parenting advice. We're all just walking this path together, each of us and our children, hand in hand.

Will this book be a quick-fix manual with overnight solutions? No, but I do hope it offers some insight, guidance, and more importantly, that it gives you a whole lot of permission.

Permission to not be perfect. Permission to be human. And permission to find your own way.

HOW TO USE THIS BOOK

The book is organized like the natural cycle of a wave or the shape of a mountain. In fact, we see this life cycle over and over again in nature, whether it be the phases of the moon or the changing of the seasons (even labor contractions and toddler tantrums follow the same pattern): a slow beginning, a cresting middle, and a quiet end, before repeating again.

Every chapter is themed around a yoga-based concept and includes a yoga pose to support the teachings. After the posture, we will deep dive into the yoga-based wisdom and explore different psychological principles and research, learning how these concepts apply to parenting.

In addition to the opening posture, each chapter contains:

- "Breath Breaks": invitations to mindfully breathe.
- "On the Mat": practices to show us how we can apply the lessons on our yoga mat in a more general sense.
- "Parenting in Practice": offerings and advice from parents in the United States and abroad.
- "Off the Mat and into the Family": fun exercises to help us bring the work off the mat and into our homes.

You will need your yoga mat, but I also recommend having a pen and journal (or your smartphone!) nearby to write alongside this book. I have summarized each chapter into some main points called "Ten Takeaways for Busy Parents" for those of us who struggle to finish an entire chapter or who just need a refresher afterward. I have also included a comprehensive Resources section at the end of the book.

At the very end of the book, all the poses will be woven together into a single "Yoga of Parenting Sequence" so that we can reinforce each of the lessons explored and insights gained in our physical bodies.

I have learned so much from all the experts and parents I got to speak with. Everyone is so uniquely different, and everyone's families and perspectives are so uniquely different, but everyone has the same intention: love and connection.

I'm honored to weave together the millennia of collective wisdom that yogic texts, science-based research, experts, and parents offer in these pages.

FINAL THOUGHTS

Everything you need to know is inside of you. This book will not transform you into a great parent because spoiler alert: you already are.

Instead, this book will help you rediscover that same unconditional love you feel toward your children for yourself.

And when you come back to yourself, when you feel connected and whole, you will be able to approach your family with a focused mind and a whole heart.

This is yoga.

This is parenthood.

Grab your mat and your journal. Let's begin. . . .

PART ONE

Awareness

1

To Raise a Life, You Need Life-Force Energy

Do not ask your children to strive for extraordinary lives. Such striving may seem admirable, but it is the way of foolishness. Help them instead to find the wonder and the marvel of an ordinary life. Show them the joy of tasting tomatoes, apples, and pears. Show them how to cry when pets and people die. Show them the infinite pleasure in the touch of a hand. And make the ordinary come alive for them. The extraordinary will take care of itself.

—William Martin, *The Parent's Tao Te Ching*

.....

Constructive Rest Pose

If there is one thing every parent in the entire world could benefit from a little more of, it's probably rest. Constructive Rest Pose is a shape borrowed from the movement-based alternative therapy method the Alexander Technique. It is an accessible way for most bodies to lie down comfortably. Taking a pause to rest in this simple shape may feel luxurious for parents, but perhaps if we can remember that its purpose is to reconnect us to our deepest self—our soul—that pause can transform from feeling superfluous to essential.

Lie on your back with your knees bent. Take your feet a little wider than your hips and let your inner knees come together. Find a comfortable distance for your hip joints and lower back.

Take your arms out to the sides shoulder-height and bend your elbows so your palms face skyward.

Begin by simply observing your body and its contact with the floor. Feel the soles of your feet, the back of your pelvis, your rib cage, the backs of your arms, and the back of your head.

Let your bones become heavy, as if the earth could envelop you.

Now, notice your breath. What is your natural pattern? Without changing anything, simply watch where and how you are breathing. Observe without judgment.

As you watch your breath, as you become conscious of your patterns, does your breath begin to shift? Does it automatically become deeper, like an A student trying to win your attention? Or does it become slower and shallower, like a shy mouse?

Simply observe.

Start taking fuller, more conscious breaths by inhaling from the lowest part of your belly up into the chest. Pause and then softly exhale the breath. Pause here at the end before refilling with another breath.

Observe for ten full breaths.

Please note, if watching or manipulating your breath is triggering or frustrating for you, simply remain focused on the sensation of your body on the floor instead.

Hug your knees into your chest, roll to a side, and press up to sitting.

Before we begin, simply pause.

.....

LIVING ON AN EXHALE

For someone who teaches breath awareness for a living, I probably don't breathe as much as I should. Or at least, I don't really inhale. My entire life seems to occur on the power of an exhale. I push forward, I give everything my all, and then wonder at the end of the day why I'm exhausted. It was getting pregnant with my first child, Jonah, when I truly started to understand the importance of the inhale; of making sure to schedule things that fill *my* tank just as much as I liked to empty it all out for others.

Sure, I would preach to yoga students about the necessities of self-care and write the typical weekly social media post advocating for it (candles, hashtag, and all), but for most of my adult life, I would overwork and overplan and overdo because I thought that was what I had to do to make people happy. Plus, the only person who ever paid for it was me.

When I got married and started having children, I began to see the effects that my choices had on the entire family system. If I am burned out or empty, I get short with my husband. I get overstimulated by everything my children do. I have difficulty sleeping and am constantly on edge, despite being incredibly tired. I get sick and sometimes I even injure myself.

At first, I was confused. I thought giving everyone and everything my all was the most mom-like thing I could do. I mean, we all read Shel Silverstein's *The Giving Tree* as children, right? But as I continually hit these patches of severe burnout and let my energy tank get down to fumes, I realized that there is nothing selfless about giving yourself entirely to others.

How can you give life if your life force is depleted?

The short answer: you can't.

Remember the heart of the word *yoga*? Yoga is about union and connection, and while of course it is important to be unified and connected to our bodies and our breath, what of our connection to self?

Putting our needs aside does not make us better parents. The more disconnected we are from ourselves, the more disconnected we are from everyone else. It is impossible to be fully present with someone when you cannot be fully present with yourself. It is impossible to give someone your all if you have nothing to give.

In order to exhale, we must first inhale. In order to play, we need to rest. In order to spend quality time with those we love, we need alone time. We sometimes need to step back to lean in. We sometimes need to say no to say yes.

We must do the things that fill *us* up or we will have nothing to give.

YOGA, LIFE FORCE, AND THE BREATH

The breath is often said to be the gateway to our body, our mind, our life force, and some even believe, our soul. One of the things that differentiates asana, the physical practice of yoga, from other types of movement is the use of the breath to both access and still the mind.

The breath can be one of the first indicators of our reactivity or energy levels. When we get worked up or upset with our kids, we may hold our breath or breathe shallowly. Changing our breath can change our life (and our family life). To the point that a 2018 study in the *Frontiers of Human Neuroscience* journal is matter-of-factly titled "How Breath Control Can Change Your Life." This study found slow breathing to be significantly correlated to psychological well-being, a balanced nervous system, and emotional control. Many other well-designed and peer-reviewed studies confirm as well that our breath is intricately related to our stress levels—the better we breathe, the less stressed we tend to be, and vice versa.

In the yoga tradition, breath is much more than just oxygen fueling our lungs and blood. Breath is our link to our prana, our vital life-force energy. In the Chandogya Upanishad, verses 5.1.6-15, we find the story "Quarrel Among the Senses" in which the senses speech, sight, hearing, the mind, and prana are all trying to figure out who is the "superior sense." As the story goes, each "sense" starts to leave the body one by one to see the effects of its absence. They are all surprised that the body can continue even when unable to speak, see, hear, or think, but when prana is about to leave, all the other senses beg it not to and bow down in reverence, realizing that without breath, without vital life-force energy, we are empty.

I teach vinyasa flow and for over a decade I practiced Mysore-style Ashtanga yoga. These are breath-based practices where movements and counts are set to particular breaths. For example, in vinyasa flow, you lift your arms on an inhale and then lower them on an exhale. Or in Mysore-style Ashtanga, you measure the length that you hold a posture based on the number of breaths. Some people translate the word *vinyasa* to mean "breath-linked movement," but the literal translation is actually much deeper than simply moving with breath.

Vinyasa means "to place in a special way," with *vi* meaning "in a special way" and *nyasa* meaning "to place." I appreciate this definition because while I love flow-based practices and find the breath to be an important tool to calm me on my mat (and during toddler meltdowns), what vinyasa has really taught me is how to be intentional about my choices, especially when it comes to parenting. It has taught me how to tune in to my energy and rhythms, as well as my family's. The breath is simply a metronome to help me slow things down enough so that I can become aware of my internal needs and energy levels.

PRANA IS SO MUCH MORE THAN BREATH

Matthew Sanford has had the privilege of teaching yoga to a variety of people and bodies. As he likes to say, "I've never taught yoga to someone who does not have a spine."

Matthew went through long periods of being disconnected from his breath and his body, having been paralyzed from the chest down since the age of thirteen. It was through starting yoga asana that Matthew reconnected to the parts of his body that had gone silent. He could feel the prana coursing through his paralyzed limbs from their contact with the floor, his own hands, or his teacher.

While there are many asana teachers that say the breath is the gateway to the practice, through his own body and the experience of the thousands upon thousands of students whom he has taught, Matthew observes that not everyone can easily access their breath. In fact, he finds that for students who have physical limitations or neurological deficits, trying to breathe into areas where they are misaligned may actually cause more misalignment. Luckily, yoga helped Matthew find another way to move prana. Matthew likes to say that you are in the "river of prana" with his adaptive yoga classes, observing that prana is sometimes even more palpable when moving through disabled bodies than non-disabled ones.

As Matthew regularly references in his book *Waking: A Memoir of Trauma and Transcendence*, there are many reasons why we disconnect from our bodies. It could be due to a physical injury or linked to our mental health. It could be because you just had a baby and are finding yourself again. It could be because every day that you turn on the news, there seems to be a different historic crisis and you question your children's future. It could be because your teenager has been incredibly difficult lately and each interaction leaves you angry and hurt. All of us disconnect from our bodies at some time or another and an emphasis on breath may be triggering or frustrating.

Though you will see that I offer Breath Breaks throughout the book, let this be a gentle reminder that for many, prana may need to be accessed by a different means. For example, embodiment is a powerful way to access prana. Like, literally feeling the sensations of your body as you press your foot into the earth or hold your child's hand. Prana can also be accessed by the environs around you, like when you are camping or in the woods and sense the life force of the trees in your bones.

The breath is just one mode to accessing the powerful life force coursing within us and throughout the rest of the world.

....

PARENTING IN PRACTICE
Paul's Story

Paul has had the privilege of experiencing prana both in its abundance and also in its absence. He has felt his own life force depleting when he was on the wrong career path and running himself ragged to follow a dream that was no longer viable. He has experienced a surge of prana when teaching a packed room of people all moving in unison to the sound of his voice and the strum of his guitar. He experienced expansion when he and his family moved permanently to Bali, Indonesia. The entire world seemed to open up to him, including master yoga teachers, yoga teaching jobs, and even exposure to different parenting styles. He also experienced the tamping down of Bali's life force when the global shutdowns of March 2020 led many businesses on the island to shut down or shutter, nearly decimating Indonesia's economy and leaving Paul without work for many months.

But when Paul experienced prana in its purest form was when his son was born. Meeting this new life was the most spaciousness he had ever felt. As Paul recalls, "He truly is the happy baby, unless he's hungry or tired."

Watching his son grow and develop each week has become its own kind of yoga practice, its own bath in the river of prana. There's no more powerful meditation than eye-gazing together at four o'clock in the morning, when only the two of them and the birds are awake. The whole universe seems to exude from this child, and with good reason. Children are pure consciousness. They are living, breathing reminders of all of our true nature: love and expansion.

....

ON THE MAT

What is your experience when a teacher asks you to tune in to your breath? Is it an easy pathway for you? Or does it feel suffocating and inaccessible? Try this: feel into whatever is in contact with the floor right now as you read this. If you are standing, it will be your feet. If you are sitting, it will be your sit bones. If you are lying on your tummy, it will be your pubic bone and lower ribs. Imagine that whatever you are pressing down into—the carpet, the hardwood, your mat, your bed—is rebounding back up into your body. Like Newton's Third Law states, "Every action has an opposite and equal reaction." Many translate this to mean, "What goes down must come up" or in yoga asana, we often say, "Root to rise." Do you feel an energy rising into you when you press down into the ground below? Is there a reaction to your action? This is prana.

LA PAUSE

There are a number of powerful reasons why yoga practitioners work with breath, from moving pranic energy to finding lightness and space, but as a parent, a big benefit of taking a breath has less to do with the oxygen we are bringing into our lungs and much more to do with the pause it allows between our reactions and responses.

In her hilarious and insightful book *Bringing up Bébé: One American Mother Discovers the Wisdom of French Parenting*, the author Pamela Druckerman shares with American parents an invaluable parenting tool. In France, she observes that many French babies are "doing their nights" (sleeping through the night) from as early as six weeks after birth! Meanwhile her American child is up at all hours and, as a result, keeping the entire building and *rue* awake.

What Druckerman unearths after speaking with a variety of French parents and childhood experts is that there is an unspoken concept in France she coins "La Pause." French parents spend a lot of time first observing their newborn's "natural rhythms" before jumping in to act. For example, French parents patiently wait for anywhere from five to ten minutes rather than immediately tending to a baby upon any noise or rousing, which often enables the baby to either self-soothe back to sleep or for the parent to confirm that they weren't awake in the first place.

Newborns' sleep cycles are much shorter than adults'. The average adult sleep cycle is ninety minutes, while an average newborn sleep cycle can range anywhere from thirty minutes to an hour. For the first six months of their lives (plus or minus), babies have a very hard time connecting those cycles. This is because they spend much more time in the REM stage of sleep. This phase is associated with memory consolidation and dreaming, and as such, our brain activity is high and the phase is considered light sleep.

This is why babies often wake up crying or sleep-cry, but as Druckerman warns, "If a parent automatically interprets this cry as a demand for food or a sign of distress and rushes in to soothe the baby, the baby will have a hard time learning to connect the cycles on his own. That is, he'll need an adult to come in and soothe him back to sleep at the end of each cycle."

We wake up throughout the night too as adults; we just don't remember as we're able to link our sleep cycles together.

The pause recommendation is an invaluable tool for parents of infants, but we can actually use the model of La Pause throughout our children's lives. As our children get older, our impulse to jump in and help before they have had time to figure it out themselves does not go away. Instead, our urge to step in and save the day just shifts to the bigger challenges they face, like when they are struggling with schoolwork or friends. We end up trying to problem-solve for them.

La Pause can remind us that taking a deep breath is really about taking a moment and leaving space for our children to try to figure things out on their own. We can lovingly observe from the sidelines and jump in if absolutely necessary, but when we leave space for them to figure things out on their own, we get to witness the light bulbs exploding within them; the prana lighting up in each cell.

Matthew Sanford tries to practice his own version of La Pause in both his yoga classes and with his parenting. He emphasizes the importance of "investing in people's resiliency versus their fragility." Meaning, we should try to let go of any preconceived notions of how things should be or our expectations of how people should behave and instead trust in a person's process of discovery. As Sanford admits, it's really hard with parenting because there are so many things we feel the need to protect our children from, but by practicing letting go, we can actually empower our children to discover their own strength and solutions.

How many discoveries could our children uncover on their own if we just paused?

La Sleep for Parents of Younger Children

You can't force a child (or anyone, yourself included!) to sleep. Yet, many of us find ourselves fighting to get our children to sleep from when they are newborns until they are well into preschool. Susan Bordon, a licensed psychotherapist, lactation education counselor, certified childbirth educator, and the founder of Kinspace, the Bay Area's premier "modern parenting village," recommends taking a different approach. She believes that letting young children spend quiet time by themselves can help emphasize the value of rest—of La Pause—over the oft-elusive goal of sleep. Bordon believes that if our little ones aren't protesting, then whatever they do in their bed is "their business."

The advent of video monitors (of which we had not one but two over Jonah's crib, for whatever reason) has made this approach confusing for parents. You see your kid awake and babbling and your instinct is to go in the room and get them, but that time by themselves can be invaluable. It is an opportunity for growth and learning.

Of course, going against our impulse to save the day can be challenging. We want to do everything we can to take care of our children and keep them happy, but are they really unhappy if they are in their bed, experimenting and playing? Bordon likes to have the parents she works with ask themselves, "Is there a way for me to back out of this process a little so that my baby can have the experience of learning and playing independently with confidence?" She calls this parenting practice "raising the bar by doing less."

Something that has been immensely helpful for us in our household is shifting our language away from saying "nap time" and instead referring to it as "quiet time." When Jonah first started skipping naps, we would come into his room, exasperated, and say things like, "You're not sleeping anymore, huh?" or, "No more naps?" So we changed the script entirely.

Now, if he decides to spend his nap hour resting or singing or doing gymnastics (his "business," remember?), we try to say things like, "How was your quiet time?" or "Do you feel rested?" By valuing La Pause, we remove the emphasis off our needing him to sleep and instead focus on him getting rest, important skills at any age.

La Play for Parents of Younger Children

Bordon has observed a bonus side to this La Pause approach as well. Letting our children take the lead on how they want to spend their time, quiet or otherwise, also removes us from having to be their 24/7 cruise director, or as Bordon calls it in her Mama + Babe groups, the family's "Director of Play." A lot of parents feel it is their responsibility to keep their children constantly entertained, but it is in the space between activity and play, often when one is alone (and frankly, bored), that creativity arises.

In addition to learning how to implement La Pause when it comes to dictating *what* our kids should play with, we can also apply this practice when we feel the urge to show them *how* to play. La Pause is a helpful way to curb the understandable impulse to show our children the "correct" way to do things. According to Bordon and other childhood development experts, parents who always jump in to show their children the "right" way to do something may actually be robbing their littles of the opportunity of discovery. Bordon explains, "Adults may be goal oriented, but babies and young kids are actually process oriented."

Stepping back to let our children figure things out can also be a way to manage our own vital life-force energy. It gets exhausting for parents to have to constantly entertain their littles. Instead, this La Pause approach to play can give the power of imagination and the joy of accomplishment back to the child.

FROM MAT TO FAMILY

This is just a reminder that the breathing exercises throughout this book are merely opportunities to take a moment, to get present, and pause, and while I hope you carry this book around everywhere with you and read it all over and over, one day, you will put it away. At that point, you'll want to integrate the lessons we have discussed into your life. This is where these "From the Mat to Family" exercises come in. They are tangible (and hopefully, fun) ways to absorb the teachings from each chapter.

This first exercise will be simple, but that doesn't mean it won't be challenging.

What hours are you generally awake during the day? Set a (calming) alarm at the top of each hour. You can just set the next time up when done with that particular session, or if you're like me and prefer everything organized, you can set up the entire day upon waking. For one full minute every hour that you are awake, for one full day, simply pause and breathe.

If you are in transit when the alarm goes off or hanging out with your child, use your senses to anchor you in the present moment, wherever that may be for one full minute. This can include playing make-believe with your kid.

This exercise may feel tedious at first, especially if alarms annoy you (thankfully, there are some peaceful ringtones to choose from these days), but our goal over time will be to try to remember to consciously pause and breathe often without the aid of the clock.

At the end of the day, reflect on the effects of the pauses and also the circumstances that helped you pause best. Do you prefer being alone? Do you need to close your eyes or stop moving? Do you do better in motion?

Parents often think we need to do these hour-long practices or proper meditation sits to do our yoga "practice" and assume they are letting their yoga practice lapse because they haven't come to the mat recently, but yoga is so much more about how we are living off the mat than what we're doing when on one.

Getting grounded and present in whatever you are doing is yoga.

Parenting is yoga.

Ten Takeaways for Busy Parents

- Prana is much more than just our breath. It is our vital life force and can be accessed through many different means.
- As parents, we must do things that fill *us* up or we will have nothing to give.
- According to the Chandogya Upanishad, prana is our supreme sense.
- The literal meaning of *vinyasa* is "to place in a special way." It is the practice of being intentional with our thoughts and choices.
- "Taking a breath" is less about bringing oxygen into your body and more about seeking a pause between your reactions and your responses.

- Value rest time and quiet time as much, if not more than, actual napping.
- Focusing on the breath can be triggering or challenging for some people.
- The Breath Breaks throughout the book are optional and simply an invitation to get still however works best for you.
- Try to set time throughout your day to simply pause, feel into your body, and breathe.
- Parenting is yoga.

2

The Greatest Gift We Can Give Our Children

Parenting isn't about what our child does, but about how we respond. In fact, most of what we call parenting doesn't take place between a parent and child but within the parent.

—Dr. Laura Markham, *Peaceful Parent, Happy Kids*

.....

Tadasana (Mountain Pose)/ Samasthiti (Even-Standing Pose)

In the Ashtanga yoga system, we call *Tadasana* (Mountain Pose) *Samasthiti*, Even-Standing Pose. *Sama* comes from the same root as the English word "same." This is not only our intention with our bodies in this pose, as we try to make everything as symmetrical as possible from front to back and side to side, but also the quality of our thoughts and attention. When the body gets still, so it seems can the mind. This pose is also thought to be a blueprint for all other postures, much like we need presence as a blueprint before any other action we take in parenthood.

Stand at the top of your mat. Your feet can be together or hip-width for stability. Spread your toes and press into all four corners of your feet.

Press your top thighs back as you lift your frontal hip bones up toward the ceiling, lengthening your lower back.

Knit your lower ribs together and broaden your collarbones.

There is a classical variation where you release your arms by your sides, but for today's work, bring your hands to prayer at your chest. Let the touch of your palms anchor you into your body and the moment. Relax your upper shoulders away from your ears.

Keep your chin level to the floor and the crown of your head lifting upward toward the ceiling.

You may close your eyes or look down toward your heart.

Hold and count your breath for twenty breaths.

·····

PRESENCE IS A GIFT

As a writer, I am fascinated when two similar-looking words have seemingly unrelated definitions. One such relationship is that of the words *presence*, as in being physically in a room with someone, and *present*, as in a gift. Both come from the same Latin word *praeësse*. I guess this quote by the American cartoonist Bil Keane is more than just a cute coffee-mug saying: "Yesterday is history. Tomorrow is mystery. Today is a gift from God, which is why they call it the present."

I would venture to say that every parent understands the

importance of presence on a surface level. You would be hard-pressed to find someone who wished they were less present with their family (although maybe they wished their family were a bit less present with them. Um, especially when trying to go to the bathroom). But let's be real: being 100 percent present all the time is not only challenging when you are trying to keep a household going but it is also oftentimes downright impossible.

I can't tell you how many times I have been cuddling or playing with one of my sons but my mind was completely elsewhere, thinking about the other kid or work or what needs to get done around the house. Just the other day, I only had a few minutes with my toddler before his dad was going to drive him to day care. I knew our time was limited and I was enjoying his company, yet I found myself clock-watching, itching to get back to my writing. At one point, I missed half of a story he had been telling because I was brainstorming an assignment. And I teach presence for a living!

I find my mind wandering every single day. Before I developed a dedicated yoga practice, I may not have even noticed, but now I catch myself much more quickly. Getting still on my mat has helped me become aware of how defocused my attention off the mat often is.

It was shocking at first to realize how little time I spent on one thought. I remember walking around a supermarket in the early days of my practice, fresh out of an asana class and suddenly feeling as though my brain was like the dog, Dug, from the animated Pixar movie *Up*. In the movie, the dog talks calmly and then suddenly yells mid-sentence, "Squirrel!" and runs off to chase something.

That day in the store, I noticed that I would be mid-thought about what I needed to buy when suddenly my brain would yell its own version of "Squirrel!" but often in the form of "You have to finish that email!" or, "Why is it so cold in here?" or, "Ugh, this yoga mat is heavy," and they would come in rapid succession.

It felt like an assault at first. Was my brain always this noisy? When I started paying attention, I realized how little I was actually paying attention.

I especially noticed this on the yoga mat, as it is a setting where other distractions can be removed. My mind bounces from the current moment to everything that already happened to everything that needs to be done. My initial reaction to becoming aware of my wandering mind was no more mindful. As in other parts of my life, I took a more punitive approach at first, thinking, "Shut up, Sarah," or "Ugh! Why can't you just stay present?" But the more often I came to my mat and, honestly, the more often I taught others on theirs, I realized that the mere fact that I had become aware *was* the work. In becoming aware, I was being present.

At first, I would feel incredibly guilty when I caught my mind wandering in parenthood. How could I be thinking about other things when I have these cherubic, perfect little people in front of me asking for my presence? It was as if I assumed becoming a parent automatically meant I must be keyed into my children's needs and energies all the time. It is on my mat that I am reminded that it is not only impossible to be engrossed in the present moment every second of every day but it's also okay not to be.

Now when my mind wanders, rather than beating myself up

for missing the moment, I acknowledge and sometimes even celebrate the fact I noticed. I am learning how to shift from a place of admonishment and guilt to a place of spacious observation. Even and especially when it is with my sons.

Here is an example of how I practice this approach. Returning to that same morning with my toddler that I shared above, where my mind wandered mid-story, the second I noticed my awareness had left the present moment, I spent my energy using all of my tools to bring myself back to him. I placed my hands on his body and listened to him chew. Had this been a day I was disconnected from the practice, I likely would have wasted the last few minutes we had together upset with myself for letting my mind wander.

I can't get those few minutes I zoned out back. I can only be present right now, and I'd much rather use this moment to be with him than spend it beating myself up for not being fully present with him ten minutes ago.

ON THE MAT

When you are in a pose and notice that your thoughts have wandered from the moment, rather than getting upset with yourself, practice simply saying "Good catch" and then bring your attention back onto the mat. Doing this repeatedly strengthens both your presence and your self-compassion "muscles."

PRESENCE AND PARENTING

It's understandable why we want to take being present with our children seriously. I mean, no pressure or anything, but are there any higher stakes than another human being relying on you to stay alive? It's one thing to let your mind wander in a balance shape, like *Ardha Chandrasana* (Half Moon Pose). It's quite another when driving your children on the highway.

But can we be real with one another? Every single parent on this planet has moments of thinking about something else while tending to their child. Even the most dedicated yoga practitioners and teachers, and yes, even when driving. All parents and all humans struggle to stay present. Looking more closely, we learn that presence in parenthood may not be as simple as focusing on what we are physically doing in that very moment all the time.

Being engrossed in the immediate moment 24/7 may be possible for my infant, who has someone feeding him and wiping his bum. Or a living saint like Ramana Maharshi, who would go into meditative states in caves for weeks on end, leaving his earthly body to be tended to by his followers. But this is just not the stage of life that most parents are in.

From ancient India to modern Hindu culture, life comprises four different *ashramas*, or stages:

- *Brahmacharya*: **Student stage.** Children learn spiritual texts, philosophy, and practice asana. The focus is on education and celibacy is encouraged. Some students leave their family home to go live with their teachers. Age range: 12–25.
- *Grihastha*: **Householder stage.** Parental stage. Focus on getting married, procreating, and generating income. Often alluded to in various texts, including India's great epic *The Mahabharata*, as the "supreme" stage of life. Age range: 26–50.
- *Vanaprastha*: **Retirement stage.** Focus on spiritual liberation. Traditionally, in this period, one's children would take

over the family business as the parents shift toward more advisory roles. Age range: 51–75.

- *Sannyasa*: **Renunciate stage.** Note: Brahmacharis sometimes have the option to skip the householder (and thus retirement stage) and go directly to the renunciate life. Focus on pursuit of *moksha*, or spiritual liberation. Age range: 76–death.

Please note: the age ranges mentioned above were determined a long time ago and have no bearing on the age we may accomplish things nowadays.

THE HOUSEHOLDER STAGE AND *PATRA*

As householders, we have a lot on our plates. We are not only responsible for our spiritual practice but also generating income and taking care of other human beings. Presence in this stage will not look like presence in the student stage or renunciate stage. Householders need to be able to remember what happened yesterday and to anticipate what will happen tomorrow. The present moment in parenthood must incorporate the past and the future.

The goal with presence in parenthood—if you can even call it a "goal"; let's say intention—is to be aware of wherever the mind may be. That could be in the past, future, or now. The Buddhist scholar Robert Thurman (and the actress Uma Thurman's dad) explained this well on the *Good Life Project* podcast, a podcast hosted by Jonathan Fields (another dad). He said, "It isn't like you come into the now by excluding the past and future. The now incorporates all of the past and the future."

Many people find meditation difficult or are intimidated by it because of their perceived inability to get present. I can't count how many students lament that they are unable to "empty their mind" or be entirely engrossed in the current moment so they give up trying to meditate before they have even begun. But our thoughts are not our enemy—they are part of our power. In fact, there are some meditation techniques that use our wandering thoughts to anchor us into our awareness.

The Tantric text the Vijñāna-bhairava-tantra offers one such technique called *patra*. In this method, we allow the mind to wander and then practice awareness with wherever the mind chooses to go. This means that being with your thoughts as they wander from what to cook for dinner to remembering how cute your child looked for their first Halloween to thinking about an upcoming deadline at work can all be considered a meditation. The key to patra is to remain aware of where the mind is going.

Describing this technique in *The Radiance Sutras*, Lorin Roche asserts that what we perceive as wandering can be reframed as "wondering" and therefore any thought can then become like our "mantra of the moment." Roche writes, "You can use any thought that crosses your mind. Any object of perception—a meal, a riverbed, a person you admire, an actor— can serve as a portal into meditation."

It is when we are not aware of the mind that it takes us for a ride. Literally. You may have heard the familiar allegory from the Katha Upanishad about the charioteer? The metaphor goes that our body is like a chariot, the horses pulling the chariot are our senses, our mind is the reins, the charioteer is our intellect. But the rider is our true Self, which means no matter how wild those horses may get, when we are aware, we can ultimately control where our mind goes.

In the parenthood stage of life, presence may have little to do with where we physically are in space and much more to do with the awareness of our attention. Presence = awareness.

IS MULTITASKING A MYTH?

I love juggling a million things at once. I get a thrill from it, like I'm performing a dangerous act in the circus. Many days, it feels as though I am bicycling on a tightwire with my family balancing on a metal bar across my shoulders (the dog included), while writing on my computer, sipping my lukewarm tea, and trying to teach a yoga class.

Parenthood is the ultimate tightwire act. We try to keep everything going at once, but even the most skilled acrobats among us fumble sometimes, and one mistake may mean it all comes crashing down.

I used to think that I was able to balance so many responsibilities at once because I was a good multitasker; however, in the last few years, some neuroscientists have started saying that the human brain may be incapable of holding two thoughts at once. Instead, they purport that what we perceive as multitasking may really be rapid task-switching, the ability to quickly toggle between tasks. For example, when we are stirring a pot while holding a newborn, talking on the phone, and yelling to our five-year-old, it's less of a rub-your-belly-pat your-head situation and more the ability to bounce back and forth between each action at superhero speed. As if we need more evidence that parents are superheroes?

This has been studied a lot among emergency room doctors and nurses and triage settings, but I think every parent of young children has experienced triage moments. Two children fighting, as a third tugs at your pant leg. Your phone dinging with work obligations. Something burning in the toaster oven, when the doorbell rings and right when you open the door, your dog slips past you. This is not an emergency situation, either—this is breakfast. For many parents, this multitasking or task-switching-like state is an everyday, all-day reality.

Now, it is worth mentioning that some studies have shown what appears to be temporal overlap in the brain when "dual-tasking," meaning that multiple parts of the brain can be lit at the same time. This implies that there may be some ability to "multitask," but as the name implies (*dual* means two), the number of tasks we can do at the same time is much more limited than we may have once imagined.

....

PARENTING IN PRACTICE
Bryan's Story

Bryan has traveled the world many times over since he started teaching yoga in 1985 to lead sold-out workshops, trainings, and retreats, but when he had his first two children in 2005 and 2006, he made a commitment that he would always prioritize family over his career and asana practice. On a smaller scale, this meant forgoing his early-morning sadhana to nurse a sick kid. On a larger scale, it meant passing up opportunities that may have seemed lucrative on paper to have more time at home.

Over the years, Bryan's family has continued to grow and, with every shift in family structure—including adoption, a new partner, and a fourth child—his commitment to prioritize his family has only gotten stronger. Bryan's deepest wish for his four children is to make sure they all know how deeply and equally he loves them, and he believes the best evidence of his love is through his presence.

Of course, this is not easy to navigate when all four kids have such distinct personalities and needs. Presence means different things to each child, and some days he needs to be offering those different forms of presence all at once. Bryan jokes that it can be like cooking "a soup with many different ingredients" at times, but where on the surface it may look like one kid needs you more, his presence of mind allows him to read what is unspoken, like another child's anxieties or insecurities. For example, one kid may be outwardly crying after a fight with their sibling, but it is actually the silent one who needs more reassurance in that moment.

Bryan acknowledges that compassionate responses are not always his first impulse. He still gets impatient and distracted and overwhelmed, particularly when facing his own personal challenges, like when he was suffering from chronic back pain. But Bryan observes that when he remains committed to his daily practice, whether that is sitting for meditation or doing poses, he is able to be attuned to his children's needs much more effectively. As Bryan shares, "The more in the moment you are, the more in tune you are with the needs around you, and when you are in tune, you make the best decisions."

SLOW AND STEADY WINS THE RACE

Though scientists don't necessarily agree that multitasking exists, what they do agree upon is that whenever we try to do more than one thing at a time, even the simplest of tasks, one or both of those things suffer.

Do you ever notice that it is on the days you have the least amount of time that something happens to make you later? Like, it's always the mornings I am rushing to get somewhere that I spill my oatmeal all over the floor. Or bash my elbow (um, or my toddler's ankle) into the door frame, requiring a few minutes of recovery. We may feel as though the faster we go, the more we get done, when balancing multiple tasks may make us less efficient with the task at hand.

The well-known Aesop's fable of *The Tortoise and the Hare* tells the story of an egotistical hare who pokes fun at a tortoise for being slow, so the tortoise challenges it to a race. Though the hare is fast out the gate and well ahead at first, his ego gets the best of him and he decides to take a nap (probably because he was burned out). This allows the tortoise to win as he trotted along steadily the entire time.

My default approach to life is 100 percent hare. I move fast and nonstop as though I'm in a perpetual race. So, maybe more accurately, I'm like the Energizer Bunny. As I have gotten older and especially since having children, I am finally realizing that this way of approaching life is unsustainable, but it took me a minute to get there.

When my eldest son was just three weeks old, I decided to host Christmas dinner for my entire extended family. You know, as you do after suffering a fourth-degree tear and living in the NICU with your baby for four days, and then not sleeping for the ensuing two weeks. Oh, and not to mention, being a first-time mom.

As I was trying to get all the preparations done, I had my newborn in one hand, an ace-bandage-wrapped thumb on the other hand (did I mention the minor surgery on my thumb?), and though there were multiple people in the house, I decided to reach for the highest shelf to grab a platter instead of asking for help. "Super-Sarah getting it all done," I thought.

Just as I grazed the edge of the platter and started to pull it down, a huge cup came tumbling down and promptly smacked me in the face so hard it left a giant knot and an even bigger headache. Black-and-blue forehead aside, that heavy cup was so close to hitting my three-week-old son. I mean, *so* close. And why?

Because I was not present. I was rushing and trying to do it all.

This experience was a profound teachable moment for my new-mom self. Not only could I not do everything and stay present but I also didn't need to. All I needed to do at that moment was focus on my baby. I could have asked any of the ten people in our tiny apartment to grab the plate.

Sometimes in my effort to get it all done and make a moment perfect, I end up missing the moment entirely.

ON THE MAT

Have you ever been in class and the teacher offers an "advanced" variation of a pose and despite being exhausted or injured (or even just not in the mood), you still force yourself to do it? Next time you feel the resistance to try the next version of the pose you are currently in, take a breath and ground in the immediate pose first. Your body will tell you if it's time to add on or back off. Now, can you honor that?

QUALITY OVER QUANTITY

Many studies confirm that it is not the amount of time we spend with our children but the quality of that time and our attention that helps them thrive. And those same studies show that the benefits of that time together do not only take place in the immediate moment but can also even lead to better school performance and improved self-esteem in young adulthood.

Even though the science supports that it is about quality over quantity, many parents still feel incredibly guilty about the amount of time they are unable to spend with their children.

In 2020, Anusha Wijeyakumar was completely burned out. In addition to being the mother of a three-year-old son, she is also an activist, a motivational speaker, the author of *Meditation with Intention: Quick & Easy Ways to Create Lasting Peace*, and she heads the wellness program at Hoag Hospital, one of the leading hospitals in the United States. Born in London and of Sri Lankan descent, she and her husband have no immediate family where they live in Southern California, so in addition to her high-demand jobs (note, plural), when her son is home, she and her husband must juggle childcare and their work.

The year 2020 brought things to a boiling point for Anusha. In addition to her daily responsibilities with her family and career, she was also managing the COVID-19 pandemic, anxiety around the 2020 election, and processing the new heights of racial injustice being stirred up within the yoga community and the world.

Anusha felt as though she was drowning, and though she was still somehow getting it all done on paper, she felt like she was robotically going through the motions. In trying to take care of so many people, she was not being present with any of them, least of all herself. She had literally put the entire world first and had fallen to the bottom of her priority list. It was unsustainable and she realized that she needed to prioritize her self-care and mental health in order to truly be present for her family and the issues she is so passionate about.

She felt particularly pressured as a BIPOC woman to say yes to every opportunity, but when she started saying no and setting clear boundaries around her work, she regained the quality time she knew she needed, with her family and with herself.

In addition to saying no more often and setting clear work boundaries, she carved out space for herself by making the hard decision to place her son in preschool one more day a week. She was hesitant at first, worried about the time it would take them away from one another. But because she was burned out, that time they were spending together was far from quality time. Instead, her mind was often elsewhere or nowhere, answering emails while he played nearby or zoning out from sheer exhaustion.

Since placing her son in preschool for the additional day, Anusha has been able to devote more attention to all the things she teaches so many others in her book: meditation, mindfulness, mantra, prayer. In having more time to focus on her sacred practices, she is able to be more present with her son.

While they spend fewer hours together on paper, the time she spends with him is so much richer.

Another important consideration for parents is that the definition of quality time varies across each child's needs, personality, and age. Your school-age child may need you to hang on to every word of their story; your teenager may just need you present in the same room while they scroll on their phone. More introspective kids may need physical contact with your warm body, and more energetic children may need more physical activity with you. Can you get present enough to see what presence even means for each child?

BREATH BREAK

Just in case you haven't taken a deep breath yet as you read this chapter, a gentle reminder to do so. Inhale, pause, exhale, pause, repeat.

YOU DESERVE YOUR PRESENCE

The only way that we will have any presence to give to others is if we make sure to spend time being present with ourselves. Bryan and Anusha both notice that when they let their practices take a back seat and do not take time for themselves, the quality of their attention with everything else wavers. If I do not wake up at least an hour, if not earlier, than everyone else to have quiet time and meditate, I am on edge and unfocused.

By the way, you do not need to roll out your mat and do a full thirty-minute meditation sit or two-hour asana practice at 5 a.m. either. There are many ways to carve in presence throughout the day. Anusha recommends doing shorter sits more frequently. After all, she wrote the book on it, literally. Her book, *Meditation with Intention: Quick & Easy Ways to Create Lasting Peace*, offers a number of ideas and inspiration for short daily practices.

Another way to find presence for yourself throughout the day is to make sure you become embodied before doing some thing and remain aware of whatever you are choosing to do. When we are in our heads, we are often moving on autopilot. Go back to Tadasana. You don't even have to be standing—just feeling your feet on the floor and getting solid in your legs can help anchor you in the moment.

You can make an intention to sit down with your children and mindfully chew your food at mealtimes rather than standing in the kitchen, rushing to eat after everyone else. Or making a rule of "no devices at mealtime, no exceptions." Yes, even when enjoying a meal by yourself.

Karly Treacy, the founder of the KT Method, a pelvic-floor reprogramming system that strengthens the mind, body, and spirit, is the mother of three. She recommends practicing the no-devices rule at breakfast and dinner as she finds those times to be "important bookends of connection for the family."

Grounding in your car for a few minutes before running into an appointment, even if it means you are a few minutes late. Getting outside and walking in nature. Enjoying your tea while it is hot. These are all opportunities for you to get present with yourself.

But rather than me telling you different ways to get present, let's discover what works best for you.

Grab your journal and throughout the day, note the quality of your presence in different situations on a scale of 1–10.

"1" being you were on autopilot.

"10" being you are completely engrossed with whatever you are doing or thinking.

Here are some sample activities to rate and observe: feeding your children, making coffee, doing your yoga practice, getting your children ready for an outing, cleaning the cat litter box, answering a work email, talking to your friend, resting (even if it's just five minutes in your car!), driving your kids home from school, watching television, or reading this book.

Important note: *try not to change anything or go into story or shame if you observe yourself being less present than you feel you should be.* The best scientists are objective observers, and we are just learning today. Plus, going into story means you've left the present moment again. So . . .

At the end of the day, reflect on the following:

When were you *least present* (1–5)? Reflect briefly on what may have prevented that presence. Was it your attempt to multitask and be Super-parent? Were you tired? Were you rushing? Did you have time for yourself today or this week?

Now, note the moments you were *most present* (6–10). What helped you anchor into those moments? Was there breath involved? Touch? Did it correlate to a specific time of day? Did you have time for yourself today or this week?

Make note of the moments you were most present and repeat often.

Ten Takeaways for Busy Parents

- Presence has little to do with where we physically are in space and much more to do with awareness of our attention.
- Parents are in the householder stage of life, which means we are responsible for generating income, caring for the family, and more.
- Presence in the householder stage must include past and future moments.
- Patra is a Tantric meditation technique where we allow our mind to wander and remain aware of where it goes.
- According to brain research, multitasking may be a myth. Instead, our brains appear to be rapidly switching focus between tasks.
- Slow and steady wins the race. It may feel like we're getting more done when we move quickly, but we actually may be more likely to make mistakes.
- Science confirms that quality over quantity applies when it comes to spending time with our children.
- One of the best ways to have quality attention to give is to give quality attention to yourself.
- Your yoga or meditation practice doesn't have to be a two-hour process. Even just a few minutes a day of getting present can make a huge difference.
- Make note of when you are the most present throughout your day. Repeat often.

3

How to Change a
Parent's Mind

I once thought I was to show you the world,
when all along you came to show me.

—Jessica Urlichs, *From One Mom to a Mother*

.....

Marjaryasana/Bitilasana (Cat/Cow)

Marjaryasana/Bitilasana, or Cat/Cow, is a dynamic sequence that requires coordinating your breath to your movement. It asks practitioners to slow down and get in tune with their own rhythms. When musicians are practicing an instrument, they often have a ticking metronome nearby to keep beat of their time. Cat/Cow is like our own personal metronome. It unveils our breath's natural pace and sets the beat for the rest of the practice. It is also an exercise of focus and synchronization as we explore moving and breathing in unison.

Set up in a Tabletop, with your hands under your shoulders and knees below your hips. On an inhalation, arch your spine, lifting your chest and tailbone toward the ceiling. This is *Bitilasana*, or Cow.

As you exhale, press your hands into the floor and dome your back, rounding the spine like a Halloween cat. This is *Marjaryasana*, or Cat.

Now go back and forth slowly on your breath. Inhaling to Cow, exhaling to Cat.

As you move through ten full rounds, take your time with each portion of the breath. Wait until the very top of the inhale before starting to press into Cat. And wait until the very bottom of the exhale before returning to Cow.

Feel your hands and shins on the floor and your spine articulating with every breath.

Use these sensations to ground your attention in the present.

.....

THE MIND IS A POWERFUL TOOL

I spend a lot of time in my head. Though I love movement practices, as a writer and someone with lifelong anxiety, I'm pretty cerebral. It is probably why I also love to move my body—so I get a break from my incessant thoughts! There have been some periods in my life, like when I uprooted myself from my hometown of Los Angeles to San Francisco or the first trimester of my pregnancies (why does time move so slowly?!), when it feels like my entire day is spent lassoing my thoughts away from future fears or past regrets and back to present reality.

We talked in chapter 2 about presence and that it's okay and even necessary as parents to let our minds travel away from the current moment since we often need to think about the future or consider the past. The key is to be aware of where the mind is going.

But what happens when your mind slips down a rabbit hole before you can crawl out of it, like a gnawing thought or fear? The mind is a powerful tool and one we can learn to wield skillfully.

Though modern perceptions of yoga seem to limit it to physical exercise, the original intention behind the practice was to master the mind in order to discover our true Self. The seminal yogic text Patañjali's Yoga Sutra defines yoga as "the stilling of the movements of the mind" or "*Yogaś-citta-vṛtti-nirodhaḥ.*" The next sutra that follows says, "So that the Seer can abide in their true nature."

In other words, if we can control our mind, we can learn that we are not our thoughts but something so much more magnificent. It is this reason that you'll often hear spiritual teachers like the yoga philosopher Jiddu Krishnamurti or the Vedic scholar and author Swami Mukundananda call the practice of yoga "mind control."

Many are first drawn to asana practice for its physical gains, but these are just the tip of the iceberg of yoga's many benefits. In fact, the physical poses originated to keep our bodies healthy enough so we could sit and work on the mind, with the literal translation of *asana* being "seat."

I have tried really hard throughout this book to differentiate between "yoga," as in the umbrella of contemplative practices such as meditation, mantra, and pranayama, and "yoga asana," as in the physical poses. I'm sure I already have or will mess up a few times (I'm only human!), but I think it's really important for us parents to remember that just because we are not do-ing a two-hour asana practice does not mean that we are not doing yoga.

Our yoga practice is so much more than the poses. We are practicing yoga every time we remember to take a deep breath during our child's meltdown. We are practicing yoga every time we are able to calm our nervous system after we've had a scare at the playground or have had it out with our teenager. We are practicing yoga every time we observe our mind wandering from the reality of the present toward some nonexistent future and are able to re-anchor back into the truth of the now.

In most of my conversations with parents, when I ask them what their practice looks like these days, almost all of them sheepishly admit they haven't pulled their mats out for a long asana practice in ages. But when we differentiate "yoga asana" from "yoga," suddenly the answers become much richer. The Colorado-based teacher and parent Mary Beth LaRue's yoga practices these days involve hiking in the mountains or play-ing alongside the riverbank with her son. Other parents talk about doing a dedicated sit every day, even if only for fifteen minutes. My practice this week has been anchoring in the present moment whenever I'm with each child and trying not to worry about the other (even if they're crying in the other room—supervised, of course). Most of the parents who still do asana regularly talk about the shift from what their physical practice looked like prior to kids (generally a whole lot stronger and longer) to now, where many are just grateful to be able to lie on a bolster for a few minutes.

If we can remind ourselves that yoga is not about the poses but how we work with our mind, then perhaps we can be a lot kinder and more realistic about what our practice looks like these days. Because if this is the case, then parents are practicing yoga every single second of every single day. Parenting is yoga.

I often say in my yoga classes, "It's not what you are doing but how you are doing it." You could be totally well-aligned in a posture and your mind is completely elsewhere. Or, conversely, you could be falling all over the place and yet totally immersed in what you are doing. Which do you think is the more advanced practice?

This is not unlike parenting. There are some periods when on the outside, it looks like I'm holding everything together. We are all dressed and the house is clean. I seem to be hitting all my deadlines and my asana practice is strong. But inside, I feel like I'm in a million places other than the present. At other times, things may look pretty messy on the surface, like during postpartum periods or a toddler tornado, but inside I am the most connected to my children and family that I have ever been.

Let's shift the focus from the outward appearance of things—the poses, the outfits, the clean house, the clean kids—toward the deeper inward connection that is truly yoga.

ON THE MAT

Alignment can be a tool used to focus the mind. Much like a meditation bell that is rung every few minutes to remind us to come back to the moment, simple cues and anatomical actions act as anchors for our attention. The next time you are in a pose and observe your mind wandering, redirect your attention to your body and see if doing so can steady your mind.

INTRUSIVE THOUGHTS

But what about the thoughts we can't seem to control? A 2020 study out of Queens University, Canada, led by the psychologists Julie Tseng and Jordan Poppenk, suggests that humans have an average of 6,200 original thoughts a day. Some days, it feels as though I've had all 6,200 of those just in my twenty-minute meditation. That's a lot of thoughts for one person to manage, especially a person managing other people. And especially when the majority of those thoughts are unwanted.

When my eldest, Jonah, was born, I had an overwhelming feeling that something bad was going to happen. I constantly checked to make sure he was breathing at night and watched him like a hawk with everything he put in his mouth. I needed to sterilize everything and everyone that entered our home (and this was pre-COVID!). I figured it was because he was a brand-new baby and I was a brand-new mother. I mean, is it not part of the job description to constantly worry?

Then it started happening during dull moments. I would jump out of the car to run into a store and forget to say bye while he waited with his dad, only to get a few paces before imagining flashes of their car being hit by a rogue driver or worrying that I'd have a heart attack in aisle six. I'd have to run back to kiss him and tell him I loved him. Saying goodbye became such a compulsion that it got to the point where I couldn't leave the room without ceremony, and then I wondered why he had separation anxiety.

When it started coming up in happy times, I knew it was something I may want to look at. He would do something extraordinary, like laugh for the first time, or even something quite ordinary, like laugh for the hundredth time, and I would be so overwhelmed with joy that it was like my body could not contain the thought, "What if something bad happens?"

When Jonah was eight months old, I was diagnosed with postpartum depression and postpartum anxiety. I was relieved, thinking we could finally explain my wild thoughts with the diagnosis, and while they lessened significantly upon treatment, quite a few of them still continued to occur.

I felt robbed. I was finally seeking help. Why were these thoughts still happening? Well, while I had talked to my therapist and psychiatrist and support system about my general anxiety and my reactivity, I had actually been ashamed to tell them about some of the images and thoughts that would pop into my head.

Once I felt a bit more grounded as far as my mood and anxiety, I started to privately research what these horrifying thoughts were. I also then felt brave enough to talk to my mental health team. It turned out I was having (and still do by the way—especially now with a new baby) *intrusive thoughts*. These are unwanted images and ideas, generally around danger or death or of a sexual nature. Research reassures us that not only are these incredibly common amid new parents but also all human beings.

A 2019 study in the peer-reviewed journal *BMC Psychiatry* reported that 80 to 90 percent of the general population gets them, and estimated that 70 percent to 100 percent of all new mothers will experience them. A common one for parents are images of harming their baby or of your child being harmed. That's a lot of what was playing in my head. Trigger warning: some of my common ones were imagining losing grip on my son's stroller at the top of a tall San Francisco hill or picturing him running directly into traffic at a busy intersection, though he was standing right next to me. These thoughts can be disturbing and shame-inducing and as such, a lot of parents don't talk about them.

Once I realized how common they are, I was reassured by how incredibly human it is to have them. Still, some intrusive thoughts can be the sign or result of severe mental health disorders such as post-traumatic stress disorder or obsessive-compulsive disorder. This is even more reason to speak with a professional about them if they arise. Check out the Resources section for chapter 4 for a few postpartum mental wellness support sites.

But if they are normal intrusive thoughts (that's not an oxymoron, by the way), we actually have the power to shift them. Yoga and meditation teach us how.

....

PARENTING IN PRACTICE
MB's Story

Mary Beth (MB) was taken on a mental and emotional roller coaster when she and her husband, Matt, signed up as foster parents in a foster-to-adopt program. The main intention behind foster care is reconnection with the birth family, but when they were asked to care for a six-day-old named Angel, it was impossible to not instantly fall in love with him. From the very second they brought him home to when they were finally granted full custody, MB not only faced the challenges of the court and foster care systems but also of her own mind.

Each time the phone rang or she had to bring Angel to court-mandated visits, day care, or trials, MB had to retrain her mind to stay present lest she be swept away by future-tripping and anxiety.

At one point, the family was attending court every two weeks to see if Angel was going to be sent back to live with his birth family—a place where he had never spent more than a few supervised hours—or if he could permanently go home with MB and her husband. It was waiting in those courthouses that the years of her yoga practice were put to their greatest use. It was feeling her bum on the hard plastic chair and counting her breaths. It was labeling her thoughts and imagining them passing by like clouds so as not to be swept away by the storm.

After two and a half years of uncertainty, a judge granted MB and her husband full custody, but even with the reassurance of knowing that Angel is now legally theirs, her mind still plays tricks on her often.

As MB shares, "My mind can do wild things, but if I can get outside and put my hand on my heart, then I can shift those thoughts. Paying more attention to the right now helps because none of those thoughts exist in reality. That's just stuff my mind is doing."

I think most parents have experienced this trickery: the thought that our children could be taken away in an instant for any reason. That fear of loss seems to weigh over the entirety of parenthood, no matter how your child came into your life or even how old they are. But while there is so much that we parents do not have control over, I hope we can find reassurance in knowing that there is one thing we do: our minds.

How to Change Your Mind

Mantras are sacred utterances used for meditation. The word comes from the two Sanskrit words: *manas,* meaning "mind," and *trava,* which means "to liberate." As Sanskrit is considered a vibrational language, many mantras are believed to transcend the thinking mind and access the divine. The most common mantra we all know and have probably chanted is the sacred syllable "AUM." Mantras can be a single-syllable word or they can be an entire phrase. It is said that the most powerful mantras are those given by a great teacher or guru.

The word *mantra* has also come to colloquially mean a truism or repeated phrase. They are like the things we say to ourselves over and over again. When I first started meditating at twelve years old, cassette tapes were still a thing (if you can't picture one, feel free to Google) and my therapist used to call my harmful thoughts "old tapes." She would have me visualize literally "changing the tape," as in choosing a different thought.

We may not be able to stop the initial thoughts that pop into our minds, but we can at least try to choose the next one.

Jane Austin first discovered the potency of mantra in a prenatal yoga class in 1996. At thirty-six weeks pregnant, Jane waddled her way up the narrow stairs to do class. Though she had stopped practicing midwifery just before getting pregnant, she was still experiencing the effects of burnout from the years of long nights at births, which had been exhausting. Compounded with the pregnancy itself, any kind of movement took a lot of her. But as she did *Virabhadrasana II* (Warrior II) during that pivotal prenatal yoga class, something clicked.

A voice from within said, "I am strong, I am powerful, and I am beautiful." She repeated, "I am strong, I am powerful, and I am beautiful." It would be another few years before she became a world-renowned prenatal yoga teacher and would share this mantra, among many others, with her own students, but a seed was deeply planted that day.

Presently Jane is known for her Mama Tree prenatal classes and trainings. She has probably taught thousands of parents both prenatal and postpartum yoga. As she describes it, her favorite part of her role is to "stand at the gate for people as they enter parenthood" whether it's their first time or their fifth. She views birth as a sacred transition and loves the honor of accompanying people through to the other side, as well as getting them started in their new chapter, with postpartum yoga and baby-and-me offerings.

In addition to her fantastic sense of humor and tell-it-like-it-is approach, Jane is known for using mantras and affirmations in her classes. These words become the inner voice that parents carry during the birth and beyond, so while she may not physically be at births these days, her energy and voice are in those rooms and parents' minds.

Jane feels that the most sacred of all sounds is our breath. She often calls it "the soundtrack to our lives" and uses the breath as a vehicle to carry other utterances. Like repeating "I am strong" on the inhale as it fuels the body and "I am soft" on the exhale to encourage the deep letting go required as we enter parenthood. While this mantra is helpful during the practice of birth, Jane reminds us that the birth is not the end point but the beginning.

To become a parent, whether by birth or other means, is to live with vulnerability and uncertainty. She observes that she hasn't worried less about her two kids from when they were in utero, to toddlers, to preschoolers, to now as grown adults. She jokes that this is the "fine print" of parenthood, though many of us may forget to read it! It is also what makes parenthood the ultimate yoga practice, as we learn to hold space while simultaneously letting go.

Mirror Lake

You'll often hear meditation and yoga teachers use the metaphor of a lake when describing the human mind. B. K. S. Iyengar poetically explains consciousness as a body of water in his book *Light on Life*: "The pure waters of a lake reflect the beauty around it (external), and one can also see right through the clear water to the bottom (internal). Similarly, a pure mind can reflect the beauty in the world around it, and when the mind is still, the beauty of the Self, or soul, is seen reflected in it."

When the lake waters are agitated, like when we're angry or upset, the surface is not only unclear but everything beneath gets stirred up too. This includes old emotions and past triggers. The surface becomes mucky with the sludge from the bottom. When a lake is still, we not only see through to the bottom clearly but the calm surface also reflects the world around it.

Life is a series of waves, and our jobs as parents is not only to try to stay steady amid the upheaval but also to learn how to calm the waters that will inevitably be churned. Being able to return to calm allows us to get clear on our own intentions and motivations (the bottom of the lake) and to become a mirror for our families to better see their own behavior (the surface of the lake).

If you immediately react and yell back at your teenager

for yelling at you, instead of pausing first, no one is going to be clear on what is happening at that moment. But if you can step back or away for a beat and then return when things have settled with your own clarity, you both may be able to get to the root of what just occurred.

Of course, our children are as much our mirrors as we are theirs. Jane is grateful to her yoga practice for giving her a forum to honestly sit with herself, but she feels the clearest reflection comes from her children. Another mantra Jane loves to share with her classes is sutra 1.36, VIŚOKĀ VĀ JYOTIṢMATĪ, which has been interpreted to mean that "there is an omnipresent light inside of each of us that knows no pain or sorrow." Many yoga teachers refer to the location of this light as the "cave of our heart," and it is believed that no matter how dim it sometimes may seem to get, we can fan the flames and brighten it anytime we desire.

Remembering there is an eternal light inside of each of us can be a powerful practice when your teenager is coming at you with negativity, but it is especially helpful to remember that you yourself hold that same light. When you look at your child who is scared because you yelled at them, or you are angry with each other, you often can't see your own light in them at that moment. This is a good reminder to take a breath, get present, and practice your favorite mantra, like "I am strong. I am soft," before coming back together to apologize and to reflect on what happened.

SORRY, NOT SORRY

Inviting reflection is a powerful teaching tool for parents. Childhood development experts have recently shared the advice that we should resist overt punishments, like timeouts or long-term grounding, for our children when they misbehave. Instead, it is suggested that we invite our children to look at the effects of their behavior (reflect) and then ask them how it makes them feel (what's happening beneath the surface).

Most experts agree that no lesson can be absorbed when the child, or anyone, is in a heightened state (see chapter 4 for a deeper dive into what happens to the human brain during stress and chaos). When our children misbehave, if we emotionally react and try to force a premature repair, we may upset the already-churned-up waters. If we can stay calm and give our children back the power to make their own conclusions, then our calmness may become a mirror for them to see their behavior clearly. This is not to say we encourage bad behavior or let things slide. Simply, it is a suggestion that we let things settle before we try to impart any lessons.

My nephew, Frankie, and my oldest, Jonah, are exactly one year apart and deep into toddlerhood, with Frankie being the eldest. They are often in conflict over toys, or really, any object the other places his eyes on. Sometimes they get physical with each other, mostly pushing. My sister-in-law, Nicole, and I do our best not to intervene right away. We're always ready to jump in if things get out of hand, but we have observed that when we pull back, the kids seem to work things out on their own more powerfully than if we had intervened. Like, when one pushes the other, our immediate impulse may be to demand they apologize, but then not only does the pusher resist apologizing (or do so half-heartedly) but they also seem to get more upset. If we instead point out that the pushee is crying and calmly ask them not to push their cousin, the pusher will often (not always!) give him the toy he snatched from his hand. The pusher feels the impact of his choices through both our calm reflection and the pushee's emotions.

It's alarming when your child hurts another kid or gets hurt; and again, I am not condoning violent behavior nor am I saying we should not set limits. As parents, we can guide our children on how to get in touch with what they are feeling (what's happening beneath the surface) and teach them to communicate and stay calm over time (how to still the surface). When Jonah hits or pushes someone or throws something, there are natural consequences, like removing him or removing the toy, but I try not to force him to simply say "I'm sorry." Instead I try to encourage him to reflect on the cause and effect of his choice.

And this practice doesn't stop working when our children grow up. Teenagers may not be out there pushing their friends or stealing their stuff (actually, that happens with some teens!), but even the best-behaved teenagers will make some poor choices that will likely hurt people. We can use the same tactic we use on our "threenager," with our teenager: asking them to reflect on both the cause and effects of their actions versus demanding they be sorry.

Also, something to consider from a brain perspective is that the prefrontal cortex, the part of the brain that helps us make responsible decisions and act rationally, is believed to still be developing up until we are twenty-five years old. This means that for almost the first *quarter* of their entire lives, our children are likely going to make mistakes and hurt other people.

A final consideration is that parents mess up, too. When it is you who makes the error, try applying this same practice of identifying the cause and effect. Modeling can be an equally powerful tool toward creating empathy, but what's even more powerful is letting your kids see you identify and calm the storms that churn your lake waters.

By the way, for those of us perfectionists who spend equal amounts of energy overreacting to ourselves for having over-reacted to our children, the authors Dr. Daniel J. Siegel and Mary Hartzell reassure parents, in *Parenting from the Inside Out*, that these disruptions can be teachable moments. They write, "No matter how well we apply all the best principles of parenting, misunderstandings and disruptions in our connections to our children will inevitably occur. Disconnections are a normal part of any relationship. It is more helpful to use our energy to explore the possible routes of reconnection and see these times as learning opportunities rather than belittle ourselves for what we think are our failings."

FROM MAT TO FAMILY

What are the mantras that you repeat over and over? The more we can observe our thoughts, the more we realize that we have great agency over our minds. While the initial thoughts may arise without our choice, we always have the choice where the mind goes next. This is the practice of redirection.

Some days, when I'm highly anxious, the entire day can feel like I'm redirecting my mind, but awareness is a crucial first step in effecting change, and I'd rather have a day when I'm catching myself constantly than letting my mind run wild.

When you catch your mind wandering toward a scary or wayward thought, use this exercise to practice choosing a different thought to focus on instead. Personally, I like to work with opposites. If a thought arises like, "My son is going to get hurt," I try to flip the script to say, "My son is safe." This also provides me with a powerful mantra to practice over and over, which will help keep my mind calm to begin.

To start, identify ten of your most common current fears and anxieties and write them all down. I know it's scary to put these things to paper, but be with all the emotions that arise alongside the thought. When you are finished with this part, take a big Breath Break with an enormous inhale and huge clearing exhale.

First, one by one, cross out the limiting belief or anxious thought. Then next to it, compose a mantra of truth that you can repeat instead.

For example, "My son will get hurt at school" becomes "My son is safe and protected." Once you have gone through each line, take another Breath Break.

Next, grab some sticky notes from that drawer you stuff everything into in the kitchen and write your new mantras down. One mantra per sticky note.

Finally, place the notes in places where you commonly go—the bathroom, the kitchen, your car. This way you are not only reciting the mantra whenever anxious thoughts arise but by simply seeing the words daily, your subconscious computer also has the opportunity to absorb these truths over and over again.

Ten Takeaways for Busy Parents

- Yoga is not about the poses. It is a practice of stilling the mind.
- *Asana* means "seat." The poses were originally designed to help us sit for long periods in meditation to work on the mind.
- It is estimated that humans have 6,200 thoughts a day.

- Intrusive thoughts are unwanted images and ideas, generally around danger or death or of a sexual nature. Almost every human being gets them at times!
- Mantras are sacred sounds, words, or utterances that can be repeated over and over again and have the power to change our mind.
- In yogic texts, our mind is often described using the metaphor of a lake. When the lake is still, we can see through to the bottom (our intentions, habits, history) and the surface reflects the world around it more clearly.
- Rather than forcing a repair by making your child apologize for a wrongdoing, consider waiting until things have calmed down a bit and work on reflecting with them about the effects of their behavior.
- We will fight with and get upset with our kids. The goal is not to avoid those disruptions but instead to spend our energy and time focusing on the repairs.
- What are some negative thoughts you think over and over? Practice converting them into positive statements and let those become your new mantras.
- Placing mantras around the house on sticky notes or in places that you can read them every day can be a helpful tool for bringing your mind back to the present moment when it has wandered.

4

Finding Calm amid the Chaos

Since no other journey is able to evoke more emotional reactivity in us than parenting, to be a parent invites us to treat the reactions our children trigger in us as opportunities for spiritual growth. By bringing our emotional shadow into the spotlight as never before, parenting affords us a wonderful opportunity to tame our reactivity.

—Dr. Shefali Tsabary, *The Conscious Parent*

.....

Vrksasana (Tree Pose)

We learn about ourselves intimately on the yoga mat. It is like a laboratory where we can observe our tendencies and experiment with our responses in a safe setting. One of the things we get to look at is how we respond in a heightened state. This seems to especially arise in balance poses or fast-moving flows. That feeling of falling out of *Vrksasana* (Tree Pose) is the exact same feeling we get when our kid gives us an attitude or we lose our patience with them. Learning what our body does and what it feels like in a heightened state can help us learn how to calm it down more quickly.

Stand at the top of your mat in Tadasana. Take a moment to get grounded and present. Remember that this is the blueprint for all other postures.

Pick up your right knee and place your right foot on your inner left thigh above your knee or down by your ankle and calf.

You may need a wall for balance. If not, have both arms slightly away from your torso, with your fingertips pointing down. Reach down through your arms to release any tension in your upper back or neck.

Once you feel steady, begin to play with your balance. If you are looking down, look forward or up. You may even try closing your eyes. You can also play with lifting your arms overhead.

Allow the rush of sensation to ride through you when you teeter. See if you can stay with it, even if it means allowing yourself to fall.

Before repeating on your second side, take a moment in Tadasana to ground and come back to center. Observe how long it takes for your heart rate to settle and for you to feel grounded once again.

.....

MY NERVOUS SYSTEM RULES

The nervous system was one of those elusive things I remember studying repeatedly in undergraduate psychology classes but for some reason never being able to retain. Perhaps because I was in the throes of my own nervous system upheaval, drenched in anxiety, severely anorexic, chain-smoking two packs a day, and so tightly wound, I would literally shake for no reason. This was when I discovered yoga, by the way.

Though it took me until adulthood to remember what part of the nervous system did what, I have been ruled by my nervous system my entire life. Having generalized anxiety disorder and being a highly sensitive person, I might as well be nicknamed "Fight, Flight, or Freeze," but it was my yoga practice that helped me understand it most intimately and the effects of my choices. Not unlike how I started to understand what my quadriceps felt like and that they would ache if I overstretched them.

For example, on the mat, I noticed that when I did a bunch of backbends in a row, I felt amped up. Or when I fell out of a pose or wobbled, my entire body would respond, as if I were falling off a cliff.

This helped me start noticing my nervous system off the mat, too. Suddenly it seemed like every choice I used to make no longer served me. Like smoking two packs a day or watching scary movies. I could hardly read the news at any time of day, but especially in the evening lest I be left with imprints of the horrors in my dreams. I also started noticing that certain people made me feel like I was on high alert, while others left me calm and almost sedated.

As a parent, my nervous system continues to rule. Being intimately connected to it helps me make wiser choices (well, some of the time). I feel it immediately when my toddler is being super resistant to something or tantrumming. My heart rate increases, the "butterflies" in my solar plexus go wild, and I need to take a deep breath. My nervous system also clearly tells me when I need time alone. If I am extra jumpy about every little thing, from the sound of a toy going off to a misinterpreted comment from my husband, that's a clear sign that I need a few hours off duty, somehow.

Becoming intimate with my nervous system on the mat has not only helped me understand when I may be going into a heightened state but it has also helped me learn how to calm down. The more I face my fears in balance poses and handstands, the better I seem to get at being able to face my anxiety in external settings. (Please note, I did not say "the more I mastered" handstand. I still use a wall even twenty years into practicing.)

I 100 percent credit my yoga practice for staying (mostly) calm when my toddler stuck a coat hanger through his eyelid (!). Were this to happen prior to a regular yoga practice or during a period of severe anxiety (when I'm in a highly anxious place, the rules change), I would have completely lost it—crying uncontrollably or frozen by what to do next. Instead, after crying for a few seconds, I got calm and was able to support him and seek medical treatment. He's completely fine, of course. He basically healed in the car ride to the hospital, and yet I have a cut on my leg from two months ago that I don't even know where I got it, but I digress.

The more we understand our nervous system, the more we can understand ourselves. While some of us are a little more prone to fight-or-flight responses, particularly if we are facing things such as anxiety disorders or postpartum mood disorders, all parents "lose it" at times, so it helps to have a baseline knowledge of what exactly is happening inside of us so that we can take ownership of how we are responding outside.

Let's take a super-quick look at what the nervous system does. If you can't retain any of the specific jargon or anatomy, no worries! This is not science class. All that matters is that you get to know yourself a little bit more intimately with each of these chapters.

Nervous System 101

- **Central Nervous System (CNS):** The brain and spinal cord. Our command center.
- **Peripheral Nervous System (PNS):** Everything outside of the CNS, including nerves, sensory input, and motor movement.
  - **Somatic Nervous System:** Voluntary skeletal muscles.
  - **Autonomic Nervous System (ANS):** Our automatic and involuntary muscles, such as the cardiac muscles.
    - **Sympathetic Nervous System (SNS):** Our stress response. "Fight-or-flight."
    - **Parasympathetic Nervous System (PNS):** Our relaxation response. "Rest-and-digest."

Please note: If you're a more visual person who needs to see anatomical charts, check out the Resources section for some more information.

BREATH BREAK

Before your eyes glaze over, let's take a breath and notice what you are feeling as you are reading this content. Do you feel agitated? That's your nervous system. Are you taking it all in, in stride? Also, your nervous system. Inhale, pause, exhale, pause. Any shift? Thank you, nervous system.

FIGHT-OR-FLIGHT AND
REST-AND-DIGEST

Our sympathetic nervous system (SNS) is often nicknamed "fight-or-flight." This is the part of the nervous system that gets activated when we almost get into a car accident on the highway. It was designed to help us survive in the wild amid various dangers, such as animals or natural disasters. The challenge is that, while we have evolved past having to run from bears every day, our nervous system has not really evolved alongside modern life. It can't tell the difference between a saber-toothed tiger, a horn, or your fifteen-year-old slamming their door. The internal responses are generally the same: we want to either run away from the danger (flight) or go head-to-head with it (fight).

There is a third response to danger called "freeze," which sometimes gets grouped with fight-or-flight. You'll hear people say, "fight-flight-or-freeze" as if they occur in the same part of the nervous system, but freeze is actually a function of our parasympathetic nervous system. A 2017 review paper from the Netherlands explains, "Freezing is not a passive state but rather a parasympathetic brake on the motor system, relevant to perception and action preparation." The authors explain that the freeze response is caused by a deceleration in heart rate, which is different from the SNS, which amps up the heart rate.

Between fight-or-flight and freeze is another place that the PNS rules, nicknamed "rest-and-digest." This is homeostasis; it is what we experience when we are calm. The job of this state is to refuel us for the next time the SNS needs to be activated.

Some scientists recognize a third nervous system within the autonomic nervous system called the enteric nervous system, which manages our gastrointestinal behavior, but for the purposes of this book, we're going to focus on the sympathetic and parasympathetic.

A healthy nervous system should swing like a pendulum between these two states. In *Parenting from the Inside Out*, Dr. Siegel and Hartzell call the sympathetic nervous system the "accelerator" and the parasympathetic nervous system our "brakes." We need the SNS to get out of bed in the morning, but we need the PNS to go to sleep at night. Where things get challenging is when we are in a state of chronic stress and perpetually in a state of fight-or-flight. You know, like raising children.

Olivia Barry is the mother of a three-year-old son, a twenty-one-year-old stepson, and a twenty-four-year-old stepdaughter, the latter two of whom she has been raising from their early adolescence. As a yoga teacher and trained physical therapist, she has a uniquely intimate relationship with her nervous system. Although a lot of us get swept away by our reactions, Olivia literally trains other yoga teachers through her anatomy programs on how to stay tuned in to their automatic responses. Of course, Olivia acknowledges her humanness and jokes that, even with all of her training, she's no meditating master melting snow around herself in the Himalayas, but she has noticed a key entry point for herself for regaining calm when stressed: her breath.

Keeping her breath calm and smooth has been the key to not getting swept up into heightened states every single time her toddler pushes boundaries, which toddler parents know can be quite often because they tend to occur around everyday tasks—like resisting getting dressed or splashing the whole bathroom during bath time or crying about brushing their teeth. Olivia has also observed that how she responds greatly influences her son's reactions, noting, "By not participating in his amplification of energy, I dampen his stress response and we both land in a more contented space."

ON THE MAT

A great yoga practice is not defined by how many poses one executes perfectly. In fact, you could be wobbling all over the place but incredibly present. The next time you are in a balance pose like *Ardha Chandrasana* (Half Moon) or *Virabhadrasana III* (Warrior III), try not to focus on how stable your body is but instead notice how stable your mind is.

Another powerful lesson from balance poses is the idea of picking ourselves up when we fall. Doing this repeatedly sends a message to the nervous system that we are safe and it is okay.

YOUR CHILD IS NOT YOUR ENEMY, BUT YOUR NERVOUS SYSTEM DOESN'T KNOW THAT

In the book *Peaceful Parent, Happy Kids: How to Stop Yelling and Start Connecting*, Dr. Laura Markham talks a lot about the instinct of fight-or-flight within parenting. She sees it as the main reason that many parents resort to yelling (fight). Dr. Markham explains, "When we're in a state of fight-or-flight, it feels like an emergency, and our child looks like the enemy."

Personally, when I'm not in tune with my needs or grounded in the reality of the present moment, everything feels like an emergency when it comes to my kids. This was especially the case when they were newborns and we were all operating on very little sleep. If my firstborn, Jonah, missed his nap, my body would respond as if a tsunami was about to hit. Instead of playing out the scenario that he would just make it up during the next nap or looking at the fact that he was not crying or irritable, it would feel as though it was the end of the world. If my husband was out with him and they were running late for his dinner, I would be seething by the time they returned. Instead of focusing on the fact that Ben gave me a much-needed break for an hour, I would get fixated that they were fifteen minutes past dinner because that would then bump Jonah's bedtime. Even now, when one of my children is crying, I can't seem to focus on anyone or anything else. And when both of them are crying at once? I tend to completely freeze.

Now, this may be a personality thing. As I shared with you all, I'm naturally a highly anxious person and I faced postpartum depression in the first eight months of Jonah's life, so my journey into fight-or-flight can be a short trip, but if you tend to experience a sense of urgency around your kids that you don't experience in the rest of your life, please know that you are not alone! It's called being a parent, and understanding our nervous system can help us get back to a place of presence and grounded reality more quickly.

Dr. Markham suggests that a good approach to diffusing heightened situations is to remind ourselves repeatedly, "This isn't a threat; it's [our] beloved child, who needs [our] loving help right now." In addition to this reality check, she suggests shaking out your hands or moving your body. Movement can help us shift from our reactive primal brain to a more conscious place. Hello, yoga class anyone? And guess what her number one piece of advice is? "Stop, drop, and breathe."

In addition to offering steps in the moment to help calm parents down, Dr. Markham assures us that when we do end up losing it (note not "if" but "when") that we can use the blowup as a teachable moment. "If you lose it, use it," she writes. "Every crisis is an opportunity to get closer if you're willing to see things from both sides, with an open heart." Because these "separations and conflicts happen daily," Dr. Markham suggests parents incorporate "little repairs" as part of the daily ritual.

RESENSITIZING YOUR NERVOUS SYSTEM

In retrospect, I see that a lot of my quirks as a young kid may have been reflections of having a highly sensitive nervous system. I never did well in large crowds or with loud sounds. Being the daughter of a music producer didn't help, but while most of my friends were in awe of the rock stars and light shows, I just wanted to get home to my writing. I still feel that way and will only go to concerts if my husband begs me and there's close parking.

I was also terrified of scary movies for a long time and literally desensitized myself to them. It used to be that I could not be in the same house as a horror flick, but I worked hard to ignore my body's signals and override them so I could sit through the entire *Child's Play* at my best friend's slumber party. This wasn't the only place I desensitized myself. I worked in the movie industry, where yelling was a form of currency. It was always startling to my nervous system to have someone speak to me as if I was incompetent, yet I thought this is what you do in this business. Not only did I take it but I also turned around and doled it out to the interns.

It was on my mat that I started intimately tuning in to my needs. Just as I had desensitized myself to be able to watch scary movies, in a way, I had to resensitize myself to life. This meant getting clear on my needs.

My needs are often in conflict with other people's. It has not been easy explaining to my new neighbors that I can't handle being in a large group of them and our children for more than an hour. Or being on constant high alert at any amusement park we attend with my sons. Or explaining to my mother-in-law and family that when they visit (or we visit them) that I can't attend every single outing the family goes on.

And as I've owned up to numerous times in this book, I may be a bit of an extreme example with some of this stuff, but I invite you to take a moment and ask yourself: In what ways have I desensitized myself to the needs of my nervous system?

Just as I have become sensitive to what overwhelms my nervous system over the years, I have also learned what nourishes it. On the yoga mat, it is stronger flows some days, and restoratives on others. Off the mat, it is time alone or one-on-one with people. And in the family, it is cuddles for movie night or going to the ocean together (without any crowds, thank you very much).

What soothes your nervous system? Take a moment to reflect on what activities leave you feeling agitated versus feeling settled.

PARENTING IN PRACTICE
Leah's Story

There is a common misconception that postpartum depression only lasts the first year of pregnancy, which is one of the reasons it took Leah until her eldest child was 1.5 years old to be diagnosed. Everyone kept reassuring her that what she was experiencing—panic attacks and feeling "off"—was the "baby blues" and that it would go away. So, she assumed (hoped) it would. Leah had not been raised to be sensitive to her nervous system. Her parents were Korean immigrants with very traditional views. They didn't talk about this kind of stuff, even though her mother faced her own battles with mental illness.

It was after moving from London to super-charged and fast-moving New York City when Leah's panic attacks became so debilitating that she finally sought help. As Leah jokes, "London felt like a sleepy town in comparison." Leah was diagnosed with postpartum depression and post-traumatic stress disorder from both her child's birth and unresolved trauma in her childhood.

In addition to becoming more in sync with the vicissitudes of her nervous system, therapy helped her see that, for a long time, when her interior felt as though it were going to shatter, she would do everything possible to glue herself together from the outside. Like forcing her body through strong asana practices and returning to travel for work right after a traumatic birth rather than tuning in and seeking peace and aid.

When she got pregnant the second time, she was terrified of experiencing the same thing, but she resolved to do things differently this time, and they were. From the minute her little newborn girl was placed on Leah's chest, everything felt right in the world.

But it wasn't magic. Leah had been doing the work every single day on her therapist's couch and on her mat and with her son, who she loves desperately. And though she has some guilt around not being as attuned with him or herself those early years of motherhood, she knows that everything happened as it should have.

Without those darker years of trying to hold it all together, she never would have realized that what she really needed was to fall apart.

....

FROM MAT TO FAMILY

Becoming tuned in to how we respond in certain situations can help us catch our reactions before they occur. Or, at the very least, help us come back to the present reality more quickly. In this visualization meditation, we will explore our body's responses within different parenthood scenarios and then, as a bit of a review from the last two chapters, we will practice employing the two powerful tools of breath and presence of mind.

Come to a comfortable seat or lie on your back. Start to observe your breath. Feel the flow of the breath coming in and out of your lungs. Notice where and how you are breathing. Is it shallow or rushed? Serene and deep? And how does that translate to your baseline emotions? Are you feeling a bit on edge? Or settled and placid? Or dull?

Take a conscious breath in and out. Pause. Follow this with another. Repeat three more big breaths, pausing in between. And now assess. How is your body feeling? Has there been any shift? Make as much sound as you need until your breath rate slows down, loud sighs or "ahhs."

We are going to observe our body through some different visualization scenarios. See if you can hear or read the words first and notice your response—before trying to change it or calm yourself down. The more comfortable we can get in that excited state, the less scary it may be.

Visualize your child reading or drawing in the backyard. The sun is out, the day is warm. It's not too hot nor too cool. Your yard is spacious but enclosed and there is a little corner of the grass where your child sits quietly. They seem content.

What are you feeling in your body right now? How is the quality of your breath? Take long deep breaths into the spaciousness of this scenario.

Take a full inhale in and a full exhale out.

Now, visualize yourself bicycling with your child to the market. First, they are side by side with you when suddenly they start jetting ahead. You are shouting at them to slow down, but they don't seem to hear you and a major road is coming up in a few feet. They stop just short of the curb.

What are you feeling? Where in your body are you holding the stress of this situation? Is it in your shoulders or jaw? What happened to your breath and where did your mind go? Did you automatically play out the worst scenario?

Try taking a few breaths in and out and maybe even repeating the words "My child is safe" to remind the nervous system that the threat is over so you can ground back in the present reality where everyone is okay.

Take a full inhale in and a full exhale out.

Finally, picture your child climbing something. If they are babies, it could be the couch. Toddlers, a playground structure. Teenagers, maybe they are at a climbing gym. Observe them as they effortlessly make their way to the top of the structure, when suddenly, they wobble and fall.

Thankfully, nothing seems broken, but they are crying. What happens inside of you in that moment? At what point did your internal world shift from calm to panic? Did it happen prior to the fall and, if so, could that mean your response to the fall was even more extreme?

Take another full breath in and out.

Start to bring your awareness back to this present moment. Feel your body on the floor and the temperature of the room. Tune in to any sounds around you and let them pull you back to now. Pause for a few more deep breaths until you feel fully in your body again and your heart seems to have slowed and your breath is an even pace. Remain in this quiet space for a few more breaths. Slowly open your eyes, if they were closed, and take in the room.

Ten Takeaways for Busy Parents

- As yoga practitioners and parents, tuning in to the needs of our nervous system is a practice of deep inner listening.
- The common three nervous system responses to stress are fight, flight, and freeze.
- There are two parts to the nervous system that regulate both how we react to and calm down from stress. These

are called our sympathetic nervous system, nicknamed "fight-or-flight" and our parasympathetic nervous system, nicknamed "rest-and-digest."

- Observing your heart rate and breath rate can be tangible indicators of your reactivity.
- Many of us learn how to desensitize our nervous systems by exposing ourselves to chronic stress and learning how to dampen our internal responses. Yoga can help us resensitize ourselves.
- Because our children elicit primal reactions and push our buttons, there may be moments in parenthood when your body responds as if your child is a dangerous threat. Breath and movement are some of the easiest and most accessible ways to calm down after reactivity.
- On our yoga mats, we experience our nervous system most obviously in balance poses.
- As such, this is a great family of postures to play with to learn how your body responds under stress and what you can and need to do to calm it back down.
- The more comfortable we can get in an excited state, the less scary it may be.
- It's unrealistic to try to never get excited or upset. Instead, the practice teaches us how to recognize when we are entering (or already in) a heightened state so we may choose to calm things down more quickly.

PART TWO

Transformation

5

When Challenges Become Gifts

> Every great spiritual teacher tells us the same story
> about humanity and pain: Don't avoid it. You need it to
> evolve, to become. And you are here to become.
>> —Glennon Doyle, *Untamed*

·····

Utkatasana (Fierce Pose)

Utkatasana is commonly known as Chair Pose, but the Sanskrit translation of *utkata* is "fierce," which makes the literal translation "fierce pose." If you have ever held Chair Pose for any length of time, you can feel why. From the physical heat that arises through the body to the strengthening of the legs and arms, it gives us real-time evidence of our own inner ferocity. It is also a pose that most bodies can do. You can do Chair Pose sitting in a chair or lying down with your knees bent and shins lifted. Another option is to do this against the wall for extra support or balance. The choose-your-own-adventure aspect of this pose makes it an accessible way for most people to observe their body's transformation; you just may need to stay in it a few breaths to feel that shift.

Stand at the top of your mat with your feet either together or comfortably apart.

On an inhale, shift your weight toward your heels and bend your knees, sitting back into Chair Pose.

Reach your arms up in line with your ears.

Be more interested with how far back you are sitting with your hips versus how low you can bend your knees.

Try to keep your ribs from flaring by lifting your back ribs up off your pelvis. Lengthen your tailbone straight down.

Hold the pose for ten breaths at first, but over time, play with working your way up to fifteen or even twenty.

While in the pose, observe the transformative effects: the heat, the beads of sweat, the strength building both in your legs, and maybe even changes in your accompanying thoughts as you safely explore your edge.

Come out on your inhale by pressing your feet down and straightening your legs.

As you exhale, lower your arms back down by your sides.

Feel free to repeat!

.....

NEED ENDURANCE?
PARENTING IS A LONG GAME

"It's all temporary" has been my go-to mantra to help me to endure the most challenging moments of parenthood thus far. The excruciating anxiety and wait of the first trimesters of pregnancy—temporary. The pain of childbirth and limping around my house for weeks afterward, unable to sit or use the restroom properly—temporary. The seemingly endless nights of nonstop tears (both me and the babies) and blowouts (not me, just the babies)—temporary. The many, many sleep regressions (why are there so many???)—temporary. The "no" phase, the pulling the toilet paper off the roll every five seconds, the throwing everything onto the ground, the hitting the dog, the pushing other kids at the playground, the meltdowns on the floor of the grocery store—all temporary.

And as I am experiencing many of these cycles all over again with baby number two, I keep telling myself: it's all temporary. I look at my oldest, Jonah, and see how much he has changed in such a short amount of time and I am able to see that the most challenging moments along our journey so far eventually become blips within the greater picture of his amazing and beautiful life. In fact, in most cases, it is the hardest moments that have led to the most profound gifts.

Like, his sleep regressions were not just designed to make me crazy from lack of sleep. They were his brain exploding with new information as he started to see the world more clearly. The "no" phase of toddlerhood is not just because he is being difficult but because he is learning autonomy and likes and dislikes. Just as the potential disagreements of his teen years will not be because he is being difficult (Actually, just kidding. This stage might have a little something to do with that.) but because he will be forging his own way and making his own decisions rather than blindly following his parents' lead.

When we take a moment to look back on the lifetime of our parenthood journey thus far, we often see that many of the more difficult times with our children were catalysts for them to become more and more who they are meant to be.

It is really important to note here that this perspective is not meant to be some kind of toxic positivity balm for us to spread all over our parenting experience. Like, when instead of listening to your real-time suffering, someone dismisses it with the canned statement, "Well, you better enjoy it because it goes by so fast!"

Instead, what if we could learn to hold both truths at once? Challenging times can have the potential for growth in the future, but we can still acknowledge that those periods might be incredibly difficult. There are some parts to parenthood that are the hardest periods we will ever face in our lifetimes, but what yoga has the potential to teach us is that our ability to endure those uncomfortable periods can lead to some beautiful gifts and clarity on the other side. This is what yoga practitioners call *tapas*.

TAPAS

The literal translation of *tapas* is "heat" or "fire." It is a concept meant to represent the necessary struggles that we must face in order to uncover who we truly are. It sees our greatest challenges (good and bad) as forms of fire, and although those challenges are uncomfortable in the moment, they have the potential to burn away the illusion of who we think we were to reveal who we truly are.

Since asana has become the main focus of many people's yoga practice in the West, tapas has become conflated with this idea of "no pain, no gain" or "feel the burn." As if we must suffer or feel pain to elicit change. But while we can grow from our challenges (if we choose to do so), tapas is so much more than just feeling the "burn" in a posture or taking so many vinyasas that our body is pouring sweat.

The first mention of tapas was in one of the earliest yogic texts, the Vedas (c. 1500 B.C.E.). *Tapas* was actually the word used when explaining self-disciplinary practices. As Georg Feuerstein writes in his book *The Deeper Dimension of Yoga*, "Indeed, before the word *yoga* was used in its technical meaning of 'spiritual discipline,' the term *tapas* enjoyed wide currency. Subsequently, it acquired more the connotation of 'asceticism' or 'austerity.'"

Feuerstein goes on to explain tapas as "any practice that pushes the mind against its own limits" and that "the key ingredient of tapas is endurance." He also notes that "the possibilities are endless" when it comes to tapas.

So, while, sure, we experience tapas from physically strong practices, like holding Chair Pose interminably, we also experience tapas simply enduring the everyday challenges of parenthood. I would even venture to say that the nonstop sounds of our children's toys could be their own form of tapas.

ON THE MAT

In certain styles of asana, challenge and heat are used to teach us endurance, and ultimately they lead to purification. In Ashtanga, you will often see practitioners wiping their own sweat back into their skin after dripping from their efforts. When practicing long holds in classes or doing lengthy, physically challenging flows, remind yourself that the greater purpose is to teach you perseverance and observe how shifting your mental outlook may affect your physical experience.

Tapas is all about fire and pressure. It is why you will often hear diamonds used to represent the concept. Diamonds are carbon atoms bonded together by the combination of intense heat and pressure in Earth's upper mantle and then brought to the surface through even more fire in the form of volcanic eruptions.

But there are some schools of yoga that feel very clearly that tapas is not actually about transforming us into something or someone different. Instead, these schools view the fire of tapas as a method of burning away all the external layers and attachments of who we think we are, purifying us and returning us to our true Self.

TANTRA AND TAPAS

Nishanth Selvalingam, a.k.a. Nish the Fish, is not only a TikTok sensation and guitar player but also a lifelong student of Vedanta philosophy and Tantra. He grew up in his grandfather's ashram in Sri Lanka, memorizing texts before he even knew what the words meant. He made the move at seventeen years old to come to the United States and study at the University of California, Los Angeles (UCLA).

Selvalingam suggests that parents may want to take a more Tantric approach to tapas. Where many modern teachers and literary interpretations explain tapas as "challenges leading to transformation," Selvalingam jokes that transformation and growth are actually considered bad words in the Tantra lineage. Instead, Tantrikas, like Nish, see tapas as a method of purification. Meaning that the intense fire that we face is not to change who we are but to burn away that which we are not. As Nish says, "Our work is not actually to grow or to heal. The work is to recognize the perfection that is already there."

How does this pertain to parenting? When we take a retrospective lens, we may see that many of the greatest challenges we face with our children are what lead them closer to who they truly are. The process just takes time and an ability to withstand a whole lot of pressure. And the clarity on the other side of those periods isn't always the shiny, beautiful diamond so many of us were promised when first learning about tapas, either. The clarity can sometimes feel like a thick goo you must marinate in for a little while before breaking free. Kind of like a caterpillar becoming a butterfly.

THE VERY HUNGRY CATERPILLAR
IN REVIEW

Quick science lesson, which you will probably remember from the one hundred times a day you had to read Eric Carle's *The Very Hungry Caterpillar* to your little one: butterflies are first born as caterpillars. When they come into this world and hatch from their little eggs (laid by a female butterfly), they are born as larva, a.k.a caterpillars. For several weeks, they have the single job of eating a whole lot of food. Following this stage is the pupa stage, when the caterpillar forms a cocoon-like structure around itself called a chrysalis. The pupa stage can last weeks to even months, depending on the species.

What is happening inside the chrysalis is pretty wild. The caterpillar's body digests itself from the inside out. This process is called metamorphosis. It becomes goo. (Remember we talked earlier about feeling like you're stuck in goo? Well, then you may still be in the metamorphosis stage of a transition.)

Once the caterpillar is completely transformed, it becomes, as Carle writes, "a beautiful butterfly."

But the transformation process doesn't stop there. The caterpillar doesn't turn into a butterfly and then is all "Peace out" and flies away. No. There's one more step that is essential to the butterfly becoming not only its true Self but also the strongest version of that self. When the butterfly breaks through the chrysalis, it is said to release a chemical that helps strengthen its wings.

The harder the struggle to break through, the stronger the wings get in the process.

If someone tries to help the butterfly by poking a hole in the cocoon, they lose this very important opportunity to build strength. Many get stuck and most don't survive.

This final piece seems to be a crucial metaphor for child-rearing. It is painful to watch our children struggle. We are evolutionarily programmed to want to help them and keep them safe, but if we remove all of our kids' struggles and pave a smooth road in every direction, they may not build the necessary muscles to survive in the world on their own.

This has been many psychology expert's concerns with the long-term effects of the "helicopter" approach to parenting, when parents are deeply enmeshed in their children's lives and do everything in their power to prevent their children from experiencing challenge and conflict.

Kate Julian, the senior editor of *The Atlantic* recently wrote a piece entitled "What Happened to American Childhood?," in which she shares that we now have "more than a decade's evidence that helicopter parenting is counterproductive," with researchers finding that kids raised in these settings "are perhaps more overprotected, leerier of adulthood, more in need of therapy." It is also why people like the 2013 MacArthur Fellow and University of Pennsylvania professor Angela Duckworth are so vocal on the importance of instilling "grit." In her book *Grit: The Power of Passion and Perseverance*, Duckworth, who is also the mother of two, devotes an entire chapter to parenting in which she shares a plethora of evidence that the adversities our children face may, in fact, help them gain a better sense of self as they grow up and may even affect their IQs positively.

FOLLOWING OUR CHILDREN'S LIGHT

Janna Barkin, the author of *He's Always Been My Son*, let the diamond shining from within her son be the North Star that helped her support his transition from his assigned gender at a young age. While she says that she and her husband were far from pioneers, at the time that her son, Amaya, was a teenager in the early 2000s, gender-affirming support for people under eighteen years of age, both socially and surgically, was still extremely rare. But she learned to follow his lead by observing the light in his eyes.

For most of his first sixteen years on this planet, he had experienced severe bouts of what Janna later learned was *gender dysphoria*, deep distress around things having to do with his assigned gender. Like begging to shop in the boys' section or to play on boys' baseball teams rather than girls' softball. Or feeling extremely uncomfortable in frilly socks, to the point it was as though they were burning his body. When they did switch clothing sections or Amaya was able to play on teams of his choosing, glimmers of his light would shine brighter again.

They seemed to find a groove until he got his period around age nine. As his body changed outwardly, the light began dimming again. Thankfully, by that point, Janna had found an incredible support system in other parents whose children were transgender and she learned about all the interventions possible for younger people. These included the social transitions of learning how to use the proper pronouns and changing identification cards and legal documents (and names when applicable). It also included surgical and medical interventions. In addition to addressing him as male and having his teachers correctly change the pronouns they used for him at school, it was really after Amaya's top surgery was complete, which reconstructs the chest by removing most of the breast tissue, that the light began to beam once again.

He went from hunched over and instinctively wrapping his arms around himself to hide the body that did not feel like his own, to standing tall and looking people in the eyes for the first time since he was little. His eyes were brighter because his heart was free to shine.

Janna and her family have always been extremely open-minded and progressive, but when her son was younger, they did not yet have the language or knowledge to understand what he was feeling. There were limited books on the matter and computers were still dinosaurs, screeching dial-up. Janna was only able to follow the guidance of two things: her son's inner light and her own heart.

Looking back, Janna feels she didn't always make the right decision in those early years. She has an entire chapter in her book entitled "Mistakes, I've Made a Few," but there were always good intentions behind her decisions and each struggle eventually lead to important changes. For example, when Amaya was a toddler and saying he was a boy, she taught him about "boy parts" and "girl parts." Now, when Janna counsels parents of trans children, she invites them to get curious with their children and to let the child lead the conversation, no matter how young.

When he started wanting to wear boys' underwear in kindergarten, she couldn't wrap her head around it at first. Again, they didn't yet have the language or understanding for what Amaya was going through, so she would make suggestions, like offering him "sporty girl" boxers instead. But after much discord, when she finally acquiesced, the shift in his eyes was profound. For Amaya, his underwear was a private reminder that he was male, even though he himself may not have fully grasped that truth quite yet.

These experiences enabled Janna to make shifts more quickly as Amaya got older. Like when he wore a dress as a flower girl in her brother's wedding, he was extraordinarily uncomfortable. She assumed it was social anxiety, but she was aware enough to never ask him to wear a dress again.

Janna got immense support from other parents and organizations like Gender Spectrum, but another place Janna felt supported was on her own mat. Her yoga practice had taught her for years to hold the space for the possibility of "yes/and." It had taught her that things are never just one way and instead how to embrace all the gradations of life. She discovered both on her mat and with her son that "when we try to hold on to the way we think things should be, it not only causes a lot of gear grinding, it may even diminish how things could be."

Allowing Amaya to lead, allowing Janna's own heart to follow, enabled him the space to discover who he truly is, and it was more magnificent than she could have ever imagined.

......

PARENTING IN PRACTICE
Darren's Story

The most challenging thing that ever happened to Darren led to the most beautiful gift he ever received. At the age of twenty-nine, Darren tested as HIV positive. The news was especially devastating at the time because the side effects of the drugs being used then were quite noxious, but Darren endured.

About ten years after his diagnosis, he was ready to have children and enrolled in a foster-to-adopt program. On the very afternoon that Darren's initial home study was complete (he hadn't even sat down to read the report yet), a social worker called to say they had a match. When he arrived at the child protective services wing of the hospital and met the one-year-old boy, named Jaden, Darren recognized this child as his son.

Though Darren is generally not one to believe in "hokey stuff," as he lightly jests, one of the challenging side effects of his HIV medicine was vivid dreams. Most were nightmares, but not all. Darren had actually been dreaming about this exact child (name and all!) for years.

It was an unimaginable gift from a difficult diagnosis.

Jaden is now twelve years old, and throughout the years, Darren has witnessed Jaden's personal challenges transform into gifts as well. Though Jaden has no memory of the first year before he came into his dad's care, it left a deep impact, which arises behaviorally in certain settings. Thankfully, Darren has taken a number of trauma-informed trainings over the years, hoping to apply them to yoga students, but where the skills he's learned have been especially helpful is at home with his son. For example, Darren was trained on how to bring someone back into their body when they are feeling reactive by helping them connect the lower reptile brain (where our fight-or-flight responses originate) to the higher-thinking brain (which helps with emotional regulation). This is much of what we discussed in chapter 4.

While Jaden may not overtly roll out a mat and practice yoga every day like his dad, Darren is confident that each time they do work together around triggers, another seed of mindfulness is planted, transforming his son's trauma into gifts. Jaden even ditches the PlayStation once in a while to use a guided meditation app.

But the day Darren really saw the effects of the work they had been doing was when Darren was bereft over the death of a family member and Jaden shared a calming technique that he had learned from his meditation teacher at school. As the father and son grounded and breathed together, Darren witnessed the deep pain of his loss transform into something incredible: an opportunity for Jaden to give back some of the many gifts his dad had given him over the years.

WHAT ABOUT US?

Just like our children, every struggle we ever go through can be an opportunity to get clearer on who we truly are. It's hard to see clearly when we are "in it." Our face can get so buried against the woes of the moment that the bigger picture may be impossible to see. The best way to learn how the challenges of life have led to gifts and clarity is to pull back and reflect.

Some tapas may be fixed events, like the death of someone close to you, which led you to appreciate life in a fresh way. Others may be ongoing, like facing a loved one's chronic illness; or for those in a relationship, the challenging process of partnership, which gives the gift of companionship. Some may seem overt, like dealing with a global disaster (ahem, like a pandemic); others may be more subtle, like the tapas of learning to sit with your toddler's emotions. But even the incessant sound of your teen watching TikToks or endlessly running around from one school activity to the next requires a kind of endurance.

At the time, we may not be able to see it, but upon reflection, we see that even the hardest moments of our lives have oftentimes led to the most beautiful gifts.

Not only can these experiences be clarifying for our own life but the more we endure and process, the more we may be able to reflect that clarity to others. As Georg Feuerstein writes in *The Deeper Dimension of Yoga*, "Genuine tapas makes us shine like the Sun. Then we can be a source of warmth, comfort, and strength for others." In other words, our ability to endure struggles as the parent may inspire our children to recognize their own strengths.

Of course, for any shift of perspective to happen, we must first endure the heat of the fire.

FROM MAT TO FAMILY

What challenging moments forged you into who you are today? What struggles strengthened you and what clarity did you gain on the other side? Feel free to look back from your earliest memories up until now or to stick with your journey as a parent thus far.

List past tapas you have experienced on one side and what was gained on the other.

Challenge	Gift
Growing up with alcoholics	Reading people's energy and needs
Four-month sleep regression	Baby's expanded awareness/ ability to connect more deeply
Toddler tantrums	Them learning an emotional vocabulary
Sitting with a moody teenager	Deeper bond as adults
_____	_____
_____	_____
_____	_____

Ten Takeaways for Busy Parents

- *Utkatasana* is commonly known as Chair Pose, but it actually means "fierce pose." Try remembering that definition the next time a teacher makes you hold it for a long time.
- *Tapas* means "heat" or "fire." As such, it is often associated with spiritual austerity or asceticism.
- In the Tantric tradition, the fire of tapas is thought to burn away the outer layers of who we think we are, revealing our true Self.
- A key ingredient to tapas is endurance.
- Butterflies are born as caterpillars who undergo metamorphosis to transform into butterflies. They are literally

When Challenges Become Gifts 99

turned into goo and their cells are rearranged for them to become butterflies.

- An important step in the butterfly's growth cycle is the struggle they need to go through when breaking out of the cocoon. If a human tries to help them, they miss an opportunity to strengthen their wings, and many don't survive.
- Just because parenthood involves many different forms of tapas does not mean we can't (or shouldn't) acknowledge when things are hard.
- The gains of our tapas are often realized in retrospect. Honor the challenge when you are in it.
- Sometimes our visions for our children are limited as far as the potential of their true Self. If we can get out of their way, we will often be pleasantly surprised at who they become.
- Tapas are individual to you. Honor the challenge.

6

Setting Limits with Love

Daring to set boundaries is about having the courage to
love ourselves, even when we risk disappointing others.
—Brené Brown

.....

Virabhadrasana II (Warrior II)

At first glance, *Virabhadrasana II* (Warrior II) may appear like
it is all about strength. But if you have ever held the pose for
some time, you may have witnessed that if we only focus on
the contraction aspect of a posture, we not only get tired more
quickly but we also may have a harder time maintaining our focus and breath. On the other hand, if there is too much softness
or too little effort in our Warrior II, then we may feel unstable
or dull. Instead, we should seek a balance of both stability and
ease. This not only allows us to maintain the pose for a longer
amount of time but we can also experience the juxtaposition
of what it's like to feel both spacious from within and held by
the strong container of our physical body.

Turn to face the middle of your mat.

Inhale with your arms out to the sides and step your feet out wide, aligning your ankles below your wrists or as wide as you comfortably can.

Turn your right leg out from within your hip and angle your back foot and hip slightly forward. A straight line could be drawn between your heels.

On an exhale, bend your front knee toward the floor, tracking your knee above your ankle.

Breathe.

Reach through both arms as if they were wings widening from the center of your upper back.

Please note that this pose can be done with your front thigh and pelvis supported by a chair.

Now the fun begins! Hold the pose for ten full breaths.

Observe the hugging in of your outer body: your front hip tucking under, your back hip wrapping forward. As well as the expansion of your inner body: your breath swelling in your chest and the intentional reach of your arms.

Observe your mind's necessary toggle between accessing inner strength and resilience and achieving softness as you explore the fine line between working hard and overworking.

At the end of your tenth breath, bring your hands to your hips and straighten your front leg.

Parallel your feet and prepare for your second side.

.....

BOUNDARIES FOR BREAKFAST

I start setting boundaries from the second my alarm goes off in the morning. Boundaries come in all shapes and forms. I think many of us assume that boundaries are just something we set with another person or how much of our personal lives we share with the world (think of the saying "That person has no boundaries"), but most days, before the sun even begins to rise, I have already set boundaries with myself, my husband, my children, my work, my family, my friends, and even our dog.

Setting boundaries is a way to protect my most precious resource: my energy (review chapter 1)—both how and where it is being spent. They are a way for me to mitigate how much of myself I am giving to something or someone since my impulse is to give everyone and everything my all. And they are constantly shifting. Just because I feel one way today or need to focus my attention in one area does not mean that I will feel the same tomorrow. Just because I feel the need to draw a hard line this month or, conversely, be totally loose about something, does not mean I will do it that way again next month.

The very first boundary I set most days of the week is making the choice to wake up well before the rest of the world so I can meditate and write. It is a boundary I set with myself but also with others, in that it means I go to bed much earlier than most and am not generally available for any outside responsibilities early in the mornings, including emails or work meetings. Getting up early gives me time to fill my cup, both literally, as in getting to enjoy my tea hot (which is impossible once my kids are awake), and metaphorically, in that I spend those wee hours of the morning doing whatever I want to do. I write. I sit quietly. I cuddle with my dog (though as mentioned, there are many mornings I even have say to him, "Not now, dude. I need a little space.").

Being able to focus entirely on each of these things without distraction or other people needing me transforms each task into a ritual. I would even dare to say that they become my yoga practice, my sadhana. Notice that no mat is needed. But just because my morning time is special does not mean that I am beholden to it. In fact, I am much more forgiving with myself than I was years prior.

For many years in early adulthood, my boundaries with myself were incredibly rigid. It began in early college around my studies and eating and quickly bled into every other area of my life. Even when I started to get "healthier," as in practicing yoga, my self-discipline bordered on masochism. I would force myself through hard-core asana practices, regardless of if I had the energy. I would withhold any pleasure from myself in the form of food or even relationships. In prioritizing my body's size, asana practice, and career, I ended up denying myself the joy of living.

Ironically, during that same time, the boundaries I held with other people seemed almost nonexistent. I would absorb my family members' pain and struggles and insert myself into everyone's problems. There was a reason I pursued psychology for as long as I did, including beginning to get my master's, in marriage family therapy: I thought it was my job to "fix" everyone. I would also say yes to commitments that I knew in my heart I didn't want to fulfill, prioritizing others' disappointment over my own mental health. Between my extraordinarily strong personal boundaries and incredibly porous social boundaries, there was little to no balance.

Since starting a family, I have tried to swing myself in the exact opposite direction. Nowadays, I try to be softer with the boundaries I hold around myself but tighter with the boundaries I have around others. I find this balance to be more sustainable when I have people relying on me 24/7. For example, I will allow myself to sleep past my alarm if I need to and skip my asana practice if I am exhausted (something I would not have dared to do a decade ago!). I am much more willing to draw a hard line and say no when asked to do something for someone that doesn't feel authentic. My two new favorite words are "Google it."

Healthy boundaries are living, breathing things. They exist along a spectrum because we always need to adjust one way or the other to find new ways to balance. There are some periods in our lives when our boundaries need to be firm, others where they need to be more malleable.

Can we be present and aware enough of what we need right now in this moment to know when to make those adjustments?

STHIRA/SUKHA

According to the Oxford Dictionary, a boundary "is a real or imagined line that marks the limits or edges of something and separates it from other things or places; a dividing line."

In other words, it means knowing where we end and where others begin. Some parents may feel uncomfortable reading this definition and applying it to their parenting. They may think to themselves, "But my child is a part of me and I'm a part of them." Others may be raising their children in very separate roles, believing parents should be on an entirely different level than their children.

There is a concept in yoga called *sthira/sukha*. This term was one of the original descriptors for the word *asana*. In sutra 2.46 of Patañjali's Yoga Sutra, *asana*, which technically means "seat" (though it is now more commonly thought of as "pose"), is described as both steady and sweet, strong and flexible.

I find these extremes to be representative of the two ends of our boundary spectrum. On one side, we can have too much sukha, too much softness, where there is no delineation between us and everything or everyone else. It's like our boundaries are completely porous and everything seeps through. On the other hand, if there is too much sthira, too much hardness, we are often very resistant to adjustments and inflexible in our thinking. Things that are hardened tend to snap and break—think of a tree branch.

When looking at sthira and sukha within asana, we can think of the elements of strength and flexibility. Having too much sthira in a pose could be like hardening, either from overworking or holding your breath. This approach often takes a lot of energy and leaves us tired after practice. Hypermobile bodies, those who move beyond their joint's "normal" range of motion, and students who put little muscular effort into poses, tend to have a lot of sukha. When you have too much sukha in a pose, it can leave you tired in a different way. Unlike sthira, when we get tired from overworking, underworking can be tiring in that it induces a quality of *tamas*, or dullness.

ON THE MAT

The next time you are in Warrior II (or feel free to repeat it right now), do an experiment. On the first side, tense all your muscles and overwork every aspect of the pose. Sit as low as you can into your front thigh and firm your back quadricep. Pull your belly button tightly toward your spine and reach vigorously through your arms. Maybe even scrunch up your face for a moment or two. Notice what happens to your breath when you take this approach and observe your energy levels both within and after the pose. This is sthira.

On the second side, barely sit into your front thigh or engage your back leg. Let your arms hang limply and put very little effort into holding your body up in space. Imagine even the skin on your face hanging loosely. Observe. What is your breath like in this less engaged state? Where is your mind? Ironically, your body may even tire more easily than it had on the other side. After you come out, observe your overall energy. This is sukha.

Now, let's look at these concepts from a parenting lens.

THE EMPATHIC PARENT

While it seems on social media that there are myriad parenting hashtags these days (I mean, styles), from gentle parenting to conscious parenting to peaceful parenting to positive parenting, most psychologists and parenting experts agree that all styles of parenting can be summed up into one of four categories. These categories are heavily influenced by culture, so just a heads-up that I'm taking a very North American lens when reviewing these concepts.

Parenting styles are often broken into four quadrants based on a parent's level of support and level of demand.

Authoritarian Parents

- Demand/Support: High demand, minimal emotional support.
- Sthira/Sukha Spectrum: Far end of the sthira side of spectrum.
- General Description: A lot of rules with very little or perhaps even no connection.

- Outcome on Children: Studies show that children of authoritarian parents may appear well-behaved at first, but over time tend to become more rebellious and show higher levels of aggression.

Permissive Parents

- Demand/Support: Low demand, high support.
- Sthira/Sukha Spectrum: Far end of the sukha side of spectrum.
- General Description: Permissive parents may connect well with their children, but they often have little to no rules. This can look like little limit-setting and high enmeshment.
- Outcome on Children: While children whose parents practice this style tend to have high self-esteem and fairly good social skills, these kids tend to have poor impulse control and limited ability to self-regulate, which researchers have found can lead to poor decision-making as they get older.

Uninvolved Parents

- Demand/Support: Low demand, low support.
- Sthira/Sukha Spectrum: These parents are not even really on the spectrum, to the point that this category is sometimes called "neglectful parenting."
- General Description: These parents offer food, clothing, and shelter, and that's it (many times, those things aren't even offered). There is limited interaction between the parent and child, and very few, if any rules.
- Outcome on children: Children raised in these types of homes are believed to be highly resilient and self-sufficient, as they have had to "raise themselves" in a lot of ways. But

they also tend to have significant challenges in personal relationships and limited emotional regulation.

Authoritative Parents

- Demand/Support: High demand, high support.
- Sthira/Sukha Spectrum: Center
- General Description: This style is the sweet spot that many parenting experts suggest we aim for. Parents and children are close, and the parents communicate well and nurture their children, but they are also stern when it comes to limit-setting and clear about what is acceptable and what is unacceptable.
- Outcome on Children: Children raised in this style tend to have good impulse control, high self-esteem, high levels of academic performance, and great social skills. Because there is a quality of independence, these children acquire the resiliency and self-sufficiency that children in uninvolved homes obtain, but their skills are born from absorbing their parent's support versus as a survival mechanism.

Because of *authoritative*'s similarity to the name *authoritarian*, many experts tend to rename the style in their books or papers. For example, in her book *Grit*, Dr. Angela Duckworth calls this style "wise parenting." In *Peaceful Parent*, Dr. Markham calls this "empathic parenting." I personally love the term *empathic*, so we will borrow it from Dr. Markham for the remainder of this book.

Take a moment to reflect: What type of home were you raised in? And what type of home are you currently raising? What type of home do you want to raise?

PARENTING IN PRACTICE
Dianne's Story

Without having a name for it or even necessarily knowing it was an official parenting style, Dianne worked hard to create an empathic (high demand, high connection) home for her two sons. Dianne made sure that her boys knew from a very young age that they could come to her no matter what, that as a family, they are a team. This doesn't mean they aren't held accountable when they misbehave. Simply, she makes sure that they know she is always on their side.

This was entirely different from the incredibly authoritarian home (high demand, low connection) Dianne grew up in. Her father's boundaries were so tight that she and her siblings had to hide any mistakes they made or trouble they got into. Luckily, her mom was much softer, which helped to balance things, but having grown up with even one high-limit-setting and low-connection parent led Dianne to worry about what end of the enforcement spectrum she would fall on if and when she became a parent herself.

Not unsurprising, Dianne is an entirely different parent than her father. She made the conscious choice to build her sons into her life from their birth. After her maternity leave, she quit her job as a tax auditor and opened a yoga studio so she could teach classes with her children. Like "caregiver and baby." The other way Dianne chose to do things differently was to treat her kids not as her property or less than (as she had sometimes felt her father did) but as individuals who deserved respect. Seeing her sons as individuals also meant they had responsibilities starting quite young. By five years old, both kids were loading and unloading the dishwasher. At ten, much to her neighbor's chagrin, she would allow them to go to the park behind their house on their own, keeping an eye on them from the kitchen window.

Trusting her children was another fundamental difference with Dianne's upbringing. But trust goes hand in hand with empowerment. If she gave her sons freedom, then she had to trust they would make the right choices. Hence, her favorite phrase became (and still is) "Make good choices." Today, her sons are well into their teen years. She feels deeply connected to both of them still, when the teen years are commonly a time that children and parents have a harder time connecting. This is evidence that just as she encourages her sons to make good choices, she herself seems to have made great choices as well.

....

WHEN AN OVERACHIEVER BECOMES A PARENT

As I implied earlier in the chapter, my yeses and nos have always been a bit backward when it comes to differentiating my personal life from my work life. Just before I met my husband, I was so burned out and overworked that my health was affected. I would binge and purge every weekend and then restrict and overexercise all week (and this is when I was "healthy"). I would go months without a day off, unable to say no. Sometimes I would teach a class just minutes after major life events, like deaths in the family or breakups, barreling through the intense emotions with work instead of taking the time to process.

When an injury prevented me from not only teaching asana but also practicing it (the two things I had rigidly come to define my entire life by), things began to soften for me. First, my injury was so bad that I had to pull out of some work commitments, something I had never done in my entire teaching career at that point. For a people-pleaser, my work commitments are like blood oaths. Surely my saying no would ruin my career and I would lose any new opportunities and never travel for teaching again.

Spoiler alert: none of that came true.

Instead, fast-forward to seven years later: I am happily married with two beautiful boys, and I can honestly say that in learning how to balance what I say yes to and no to, my career has been able to thrive right alongside my family.

Would I be deeper into my leg-behind-the-head poses had I kept prioritizing my asana over my relationships and developing a family? Possibly, but I would not trade newborn and toddler cuddles for shoving my leg behind my head for anything.

NO IS NOT A BAD WORD

It's not easy, learning how to say no to those you love the most. Some brain researchers say that we are hardwired to associate the word with negativity and that opposite parts of the brain fire when hearing no versus yes. I know many parents who try to never say the word to their children. I try to set positive limits in other ways, for example, by acknowledging what my kids can do or explaining why something may not work right now, versus just saying no outright. They say a toddler hears no four hundred times a day, so I get the hesitation, but may I suggest something perhaps a bit controversial?

What if saying no is not necessarily a bad thing? What if saying no is a necessity? What if we could retrain our brain to understand that saying no is really saying yes to something else? Most often yourself? As Anne Lamott sums up in her hilarious and raw book *Operating Instructions: A Journal of My Son's First Year*, "'No' is a complete sentence." The author and activist Glennon Doyle also explained this well in a recent episode of her *We Can Do Hard Things* podcast, saying that a big part of mitigating one's tendency to people-please is "having the intellectual honesty to know that every 'yes' is a 'no' and every 'no' in a 'yes.'"

This is absolutely true for me. When I'm saying yes to please everyone else, I am ultimately saying no to my own needs. This then leads me to feel overwhelmed and overcommitted. My work suffers and my relationships suffer when my self-care suffers.

Our children also learn boundaries through our modeling—both how to set them and how to disrespect them. I am already seeing clear evidence that my eldest, Jonah, even as a toddler, is requesting to set his own boundaries, and I work hard to respect those. For example, when we have people visit or we go stay with family, he (much like me) loses steam after a few days in and needs a break from all the social engagements. When he couldn't speak yet, he would tell me by needing constant contact with me, acting much more relaxed when lying together quietly in a dark room versus when he was the center of attention (that part of him is not like me). Now that his verbal skills are better developed, he literally asks to stay in bed some days or to stay home versus going out somewhere or being around other people.

Can we respect our children's boundaries when they request them? Can we take no as a complete answer when they don't want to do something we have asked them to do? Like physical affection toward a family member, eating certain foods, or not wanting to go somewhere we had planned for them? Where is the line between setting your own limits and listening to your child's needs?

This is where the connection piece of empathic parenting comes in. If we are in tune with our child's needs, then we can gauge on that particular day and in that particular moment if we are able to acquiesce; or if it happens to be a day when our child is just being unnecessarily difficult to assess, what/if any limit needs to be set and enforced. Remember to return to all of the skills we honed in part one of the book, such as becoming sensitive to life-force energy (both yours and your child's). Practice grounding in your body and/or breath. Observe the fluctuations of your nervous system. Remember that any one of these simple actions (if not all) can help us become more connected with our children and therefore be clearer on what our children truly need, so we can say yes to their no.

SETTING LIMITS WITH STEPCHILDREN

So far, we have talked about setting personal boundaries and honoring our children's boundaries. We have also discussed the importance of setting limits with our children. Remember that empathic parents are not only highly connected to their kids but also set firm rules. Daniel Siegel and Mary Hartzell express the cruciality of limit-setting with our children in *Parenting from the Inside Out*, writing, "Setting limits is important and enables children to learn frustration tolerance, response flexibility, and a balanced functioning of their emotional clutch."

But how do you set limits with your children when you are in the role of stepparent? Do you? Should you? I spoke with two yoga-teacher stepparents who choose to stay on very different ends of the boundary spectrum, reminding us that there is no one way, not in yoga asana and definitely not in family.

Erika

When Erika Trice met her partner, Malcolm, eleven years ago, he had it all. He was kind, funny, handsome, and successful. He was also the father of three daughters whose ages ranged from six to twelve. At first, the joint custody situation with their mother meant that the girls were splitting their time between the two houses. Erika didn't want to insert herself when the girls had such precious time with their dad, so she would go to yoga classes or teach workshops on their weekends. It also took the girls a long time to accept her into their lives and they tended to be cold and dismissive when they were younger.

As Erika and Malcolm became more serious, and the girls grew into their teen years, things shifted. Malcolm began to bring Erika into the decision-making behind the scenes, allowing her to offer advice when it came to big issues. While Erika became more involved in the process as Malcolm's personal counsel, she has never overtly disciplined the girls.

These days, the "girls" are now grown women. All of them are in college and their relationship with Erika is much sweeter. Erika credits not pushing her opinions on them or trying to set limits as keys to getting where they are now. She also credits her daily sadhana, which provides a safe place for her to go and practice showing up, doing her best, and then letting go of her attachment to the way things should be.

Now that the girls have grown up, they seem to understand what an important part of their father's life Erika is, and while they may not be calling her every day to just chat (not yet at least!), Erika loves her nontraditional family and knows now in her heart that her stepdaughters love her too.

David

David Lynch's journey as a stepparent has been a bit different. David first met his partner, Eva, in Manila in 2014, where he was leading a teacher training. She had two daughters who were four and eight, and the youngest became transfixed with David immediately. Though few words were spoken between he and the littlest that initial visit, she would bring him flower petals and lay them at his feet.

For the first few years of their relationship, David and his partner were long distance, so while they and the children would be together for long stretches of time, sometimes up to two months, it was only a few times out of the year.

When COVID-19 hit, David was forced to be separated from Eva and the kids for almost an entire year due to travel restrictions. He was devastated being apart and suddenly his "single"-man life in Los Angeles felt very empty compared to the vibrance of being a stepdad with kids.

The second the borders reopened, David moved permanently to Germany to focus on his family. It has been almost three years and the girls, now twelve and sixteen, lovingly refer to him as "Stepdad" or "Stepfather." Because their mom already ran a tight ship, David became actively involved in limit-setting, though he jokes his role is more that of a "subtle shadow figure." What has been helpful for them as a family is having set chores and roles for everyone in the house, which he then gently enforces.

But the most important boundary David has set is with himself and his work-life balance. When they were living apart, it was easy for David to be overscheduled with classes and travel gigs. He loves interacting with students, especially in teacher-training settings, but while prior to being a stepdad he may have been sucked into draining interactions or working extra hours, he now feels much more confident and even relieved to say, "No, sorry. I have to get home to my kids."

FROM MAT TO FAMILY

Let's observe our various boundaries in different aspects of our lives. Check out the sthira/sukha continuum we have drawn for you (pictured below) and reflect on different areas of your life. The below suggestions are just a few categories to get you started. You may come up with many more or get even more specific. For example, maybe there is one specific family member you have a hard time setting boundaries with, while you feel clear with all the others. Or perhaps there is one aspect of work that you have too hard of boundaries and wish you could soften.

Feel free to take as macro or as micro of a view as you need!

After you have determined your boundaries in each category, reflect on what you have observed.

Finally, what are three simple actions you can take to find more balance in this moment overall?

• ———— •		With my child(ren)
• ———— •		With my work
• ———— •		With my asana practice
• ———— •		With my partner
• ———— •		With my friends
• ———— •		With limit-setting with my child(ren)
• ———— •		With my free time

Sthira   Sukha

Ten Takeaways for Busy Parents

- Boundaries can apply to almost every aspect of our lives. They are knowing where we end and where others begin.
- In Patañjali's Yoga Sutra, we are taught the concept of *sthira* and *sukha*, which means "steady and soft" or "strong and soft."
- Sthira/sukha is traditionally used to describe the desired balance we seek in asana ("seat" or "posture"), but it can also be applied to the general boundaries we set throughout our life.
- *Sthira* means "strong," and it correlates to having rigid and tight boundaries.
- *Sukha* means "sweet," and it correlates to having little to no boundaries.
- There are many styles of parenting, but most experts agree that they all fall into one of four categories: authoritative parenting, permissive parenting, neglectful parenting, and authoritarian parenting.
- The styles exist along two lines and can be divided into four quadrants based on their levels of connection and limit-setting.

- The authoritative style is one of the more preferred styles, as backed by science and research. This style has both high levels of demand and connection. It is often renamed by different authors and researchers, due to its similarity with authoritarian parenting. For the purposes of this book, we will call it empathic parenting (as borrowed from Dr. Laura Markham, the author of *Peaceful Parent, Happy Kids*).
- Remember that saying no to something is often saying yes to yourself.
- Imagine sthira and sukha existing on a continuum, with firm boundaries being on one side and loose boundaries on the other. Where do your boundaries land throughout the various areas of your life?

7

If You Love Something, Let It Go

Parents have the job of establishing safety through boundaries, validation, and empathy.

Children have the job of exploring and learning, through experiencing and expressing their emotions.

And when it comes to jobs, we all have to stay in our lanes.

> —Dr. Becky Kennedy, *Good Inside: A Guide to Becoming the Parent You Want to Be*

.....

Garudasana (Eagle Pose) and Let It Fly Away

The common *Garudasana* transition of nesting your eagle and then releasing it back into the wild embodies the entire journey of parenthood. From the inward and pulled-in nature of the starting position—which relates to newborn life, to starting to find more freedom as we lift our torsos upright (school-age and teen years), to finally letting our eagle fly away (when our children [potentially] become autonomous adults), this mini-flow sequence teaches us in our bodies that sometimes the most loving thing we can do for someone is to let them go.

Inhale into Chair Pose (*Utkatasana*). On an exhale, pick your left leg up and wrap it tightly over your bent right leg, thigh on top of thigh, and crossing at your ankles, if you are able. If you are unable to wrap your ankles, keep your left toes on the floor or a block, like a kickstand.

Reach your arms in front of your chest and cross your right elbow over your left elbow. Perhaps double-crossing at your wrists and maybe even bringing your opposite palms together. Of course, if you're not able, you can do the variation of simply giving yourself a hug.

Take an inhale upright and then on an exhale, round your spine, touching your elbows to your knees. Hold for five breaths.

On an inhale, slowly come back upright with your torso. Untangle your arms, reaching them up in line with your ears.

Unwrap your top leg and stand up tall while stretching it out straight in front of you. This is considered letting our eagle "fly away." Pause in this shape before lowering your lifted leg and switching sides.

.....

THE PRACTICE OF PARENTHOOD IS A PRACTICE OF LETTING GO

I was not prepared for how many facets of parenting require letting go. My oldest is only two and a half years old as I write this, and I feel as though I have already had to let go a hundred times. From the loss of him no longer being glued to my chest to wanting to roll around on the floor. From the transition of him being constantly carried to now having to be chased. From him needing me to do absolutely everything to now demanding "I do it" with even the most complicated of tasks.

As the child/sister/wife/cousin/niece/granddaughter/ friend of addicts and alcoholics, letting go in any area of my life, particularly with my children, is one of the hardest things for me to practice. I grew up surrounded by great instability. It is a roller coaster not knowing what side of someone's personality you are going to get when you come down to the kitchen table in the morning. Asking yourself, "Will so-and-so be full of joy and making jokes or silent and brooding?" and then in turn, trying to determine who you need to be to not upset them.

In adulthood, this has translated into a "need" to control everything. It is how I feel safe since everything around me was always so unpredictable. It is no wonder I was attracted to a career like teaching yoga. I chose a job where I get to control almost every aspect of the environment—the music, the sequence, the temperature in the room. Not to mention that as a teacher, people do what I tell them to for an entire hour (or sometimes eight when you lead teacher trainings!).

"Lift your right leg." "Firm your left hip in." No problem, Sarah.

But you know who doesn't always listen to us? Our children.

Birgitte Kristen, a mother of two boys and the owner of Metta Movement Studio in Santa Monica, California, regularly jokes in her teacher trainings that she loves and appreciates how well the teacher trainees listen to her because when she returns home, her family does not listen quite as well.

You may say that my desire to control things is especially strong given my upbringing, but like most things we have been exploring, our need to control versus our ability to let go exists on a spectrum. You may have the complete opposite approach than me—letting people in your life do whatever they want, whenever they want, without any anxiety.

First, are you a unicorn? And second, no matter the degree or your reaction to it, all parents must face some form of letting go. In fact, we must face it over and over again. This pattern is endemic throughout the entire course of parenthood. Maybe one could argue that this is the heart of the whole practice of parenting: learning to let go. Our children are not ours, even if they come from our bodies, even if they look exactly like us. They are with us temporarily. And while we will always love them, while we will always be connected on a soul level, in human form, it seems like they are meant to leave us, in different ways, again and again and again.

It breaks my heart when I look at my sons and remember that this moment is going to pass and they are no longer going to need me in the same way, but it also helps me treat the privilege of the moment with even more respect. Remembering that every moment is fleeting helps me appreciate them that much more.

VAIRAGYA

In the first *pada* of Patañjali's Yoga Sutra, he talks about the concepts of *abhyasa* and *vairagya*. *Abhyasa* is often translated to mean "practice" or "effort" and *vairagya* as "nonattachment."

Throughout sutras 1.12 to 1.16, Patañjali discusses abhyasa and vairagya as the key ingredients to stilling the movements of the mind. Reverend Jaganath Carrera's book *Inside the Yoga Sutras* sums up these five sutras well. He writes, "The combination of practice and nonattachment leads to becoming an individual who develops his or her capacities to the fullest and who is guided by a clear, selfless mind."

Personally, I interpret this set of sutras to mean that we should do the best that we can but also let go of any expectations of outcome. When we do something with anticipation of the outcome, we are bound to be disappointed. My mom loved the Alcoholics Anonymous saying, "Expectations lead to premeditated resentments." There is great peace to be found when we can show up for things fully in our hearts without any attachment to the results.

Many scholars refer to abhyasa-vairagya as two wings of a bird or oars of a boat. This implies that they must be practiced together if we are to move forward. Too much of any one thing and you end up going in circles.

I have the abhyasa side of life down. Hard work? Check. No days off? You got it. No sleep? No prob. Pushing past my limits? That is my jam. But even if I make some initial progress pushing my way through life, I inevitably come crashing down. I need that second wing. We all do.

The vairagya of it all is a lot more challenging for me. Its root word, *viraga*, means "without color." "Viraga means 'devoid of any coloring, influence, or attachment," as Dr. Pandit Rajmani Tigunait's describes in his book *The Secret of the Yoga Sutras: Samadhi Pada*. He continues, "Vairagya refers to our ability to live in the world and yet remain above it—to perform our actions and yet remain unaffected by both the process of action and its fruit."

It's worth noting that nonattachment is also a big concept in Buddhism. Gautama Buddha was first born into Hindu faith, and there is a lot of crossover with certain words and concepts, so much so that the Dalai Lama regularly calls the two faiths "twin brothers."

In addition to being a certified yoga therapist, activist, mindfulness meditation teacher, and mother of two sons in their midtwenties, Dawn Stillo has been practicing the Nichiren Buddhist tradition for nearly thirty-six years. She has been studying Buddhism longer than she's been a parent!

Dawn agrees that there are similarities between the yogic concept of abhyasa-vairagya and the Buddhist concept of nonattachment. Much of her lineage's studies are centered on the law of cause and effect, so her "Buddhist slant" on the concept of abhyasa is that it's all about the effort and the cause while vairagya is the "trust in the effect"—*trust* being the key word.

LIFE IS NEUTRAL

Life itself is neutral. Nature is neutral. Reverend Jaganath shares that his teacher would often say, "Electricity is good when you plug in a radio but bad when you plug in your finger." The rain is neutral until it causes floods. The baby crying is just the baby crying. Our partner forgetting to pack our kid's lunch is just someone forgetting to pack lunch. These are not personal attacks. Rather, it is our interpretation of the events—our attachment to them—that assigns meaning and gives them the power to disrupt our peace.

Byron Katie's well-known self-inquiry approach, The Work, is an example of vairagya. As she explains in her book *Loving What Is: Four Questions That Can Change Your Life*, "A thought is harmless unless we believe it. It's not our thoughts, but the *attachment* to our thoughts that causes suffering." The essence of The Work is that it "reveals that what you think shouldn't have happened *should* have happened. It should have happened because it did, and no thinking in the world can change it. This doesn't mean that you condone it or approve of it. It just means that you can see things without resistance and without the confusion of your inner struggle," Katie describes.

It is the practice of learning to see reality without the coloring of our expectations. *Loving What Is* compiles the various conversations Katie has had with different people who have attended her workshops over the years. A great number of the people who are suffering and come to her for guidance are (you may have guessed it) parents.

One parent, called Sally, talks about how unhappy she is that their eight-year-old son won't do what he's told. From not doing his homework to never completing his chores, Sally explains that every day she asks him to do these things and every day he does not comply.

After they go through the process of The Work, Sally and Byron Katie determine a key takeaway that helps alleviate Sally's suffering. Sally feels that, as his mother, she should have control over his behavior. A lot of parents feel that way. This is the line of thinking behind the authoritarian style of parenting (see chapter 6). Even if you don't entirely adhere to that parenting style, there are often still unspoken expectations in many families that children should do what they are told.

Byron Katie points out to this mother that while she may *want* to control his behavior, ultimately she cannot, and trying to has only led to *her* suffering. Furthermore, she is "arguing with reality," as Katie likes to say, because though she may ask him to do these things—his homework, chores—he's not doing them.

Now, this is not to say Byron Katie suggests Sally swing to the other side of the parenting spectrum and become a permissive parent, allowing her son to do whatever he wants. In fact, Byron Katie stays away from offering specific parenting advice and instead focuses on Sally and her reactions (much like I have been trying to do throughout most of this book), suggesting that rather than Sally stop asking him to do his homework, she shifts her attachment to the results of that request.

There is no law that our children must heed every demand or be thankful for all our efforts. In fact, Byron Katie goes on to explain that parenting with expectation can be a form of conditional love. Parenting without expectation is unconditional love. This is the essence of vairagya. Not attaching to the outcome of our offerings, yet continuing to give love, is vairagya.

ON THE MAT

Do you have expectations on your mat? Is there a pose you have been working toward? For me, handstand in the center of the room was always an extremely challenging pose, yet I was determined to accomplish it. Spoiler alert: twenty-plus years later, I still can't hold a handstand without a wall, but I'm not attached to it anymore. Nowadays, I simply enjoy trying, and when I fall over, rather than forcing myself to repeatedly do it over and over, and tiring my body (and ego) out, I move on.

Personally, a major shift happened when I stopped needing to "nail the pose" and instead started to appreciate my effort for the sake of effort.

The next time you attempt to do a pose you have been working toward, rather than doing the pose to accomplish the pose, see if you can shift your focus onto the transitions of getting in and out rather than the posture itself.

ALLOWING AUTONOMY

There are several movements of parenting that take this route. One such method, the RIE (Resources for Infant Educarers) approach to parenting, encourages parents to give their children great autonomy and respect to make their own choices from as early as birth. The founder, Magda Gerber, explains what this means in her book *Your Self-Confident Baby*: "It means accepting, enjoying, and loving your child as [they are] and not expecting [them] to do what [they] cannot do."

One of the basic principles to this approach is a trust in the child to know their own needs. This includes allowing them to participate in their own caregiving. For example, asking for consent before diapering your eight-month-old or letting your toddler choose their own outfit.

Many parents apply the Montessori style, which began as an educational approach, to parenting younger children, as well. Developed by the educator and physician Maria Montessori in the early 1900s, this system of child-rearing and education emphasizes and embraces children's autonomy. It allows the child to naturally lead, often through play and exploration. One of the main principles of the method is respecting the child's choices and decisions.

When we look at different cultures and societies around the world, we see that this approach to child-rearing is actually quite common. Emphasizing children's independence is one of the commonalities that Michaeleen Doucleff finds in hunter-gatherer societies across the world. She and her toddler went to live with and study some of these cultures for her book, *Hunt, Gather, Parent: What Ancient Cultures Can Teach Us About the Lost Art of Raising Happy, Helpful Little Humans*.

Whether in the Yucatan or the Serengeti, Doucleff observes, "In general, hunter-gatherer communities greatly value a person's right to make their own decisions—that is, their right to self-governance." She goes on, "This view extends to children, who are allowed to decide their own action, moment to moment, and set their own agendas." Doucleff interviewed the psychological anthropologist Suzanne Gaskins, who observed that, in Mayan culture, a one-year-old can entertain themselves for an hour! Jonah could barely entertain himself for one minute at that age.

Observing a Hadzabe parent in Tanzania and their six-year-old daughter who never fight or get into conflict, Doucleff notices that there is an unspoken agreement of "You control yourself and I'll control myself," and she theorizes that this may be why those parents and children don't argue.

Now, despite the incredibly long leashes parents in these societies seem to give their children, safety is still a priority. In fact, Doucleff observes in many of these societies that parents create what she calls an "invisible safety net," whether that is older children or other people in the community keeping an eye on each other's children to ensure they are avoiding danger or empowering children by starting to teach them at a young age how to handle dangerous situations. Doucleff explains, "And thus, giving children autonomy doesn't mean sacrificing safety. It simply means staying quiet and out of the way. It means watching, from a distance, so kids can explore and learn for themselves. Then if the child gets into danger—real danger—you swoop in to help."

Similarly, in the RIE style of parenting, one of Magda Gerber's main teaching points is that an environment must be safe first before you let your children roam free. In our house, this means having "safe" cabinets and drawers in the kitchen so that Jonah (and eventually Jacob) can have freedom to explore while we're in there cooking. The key is to first clear these drawers and cabinets from anything sharp or poisonous, though Jonah still always seems to find the meat thermometer.

Look, I am not ready to send my toddler to the corner store to buy milk or give him free rein of the house all day, but as someone who usually has to control all the things, all the time, there has been incredible freedom for me in learning to let my sons explore the world on their own terms.

Have you ever observed parents at the playground shadowing or managing their children's every move? "Try this, Stevie!" or "Let's go over here, Anna!" "Oh, are you sure you want to climb that? That may be too hard for you. Be careful!" Maybe you do this yourself. I definitely find myself doing it at times and, frankly, it's exhausting.

I now much prefer sitting on the bench like a scientist observing my toddler while he safely plays. Of course, half the time, he just wants to be next to me and his baby brother, eating my snacks (how does he always know I'm eating something when he's on the other side of the playground?), but the other half of that time, he is free to do what he wants, and I am free from the need to control.

In Al-Anon, a support program for families and friends of alcoholics, there is a term "detaching with love." I came to the program after a family member had a major slip in their recovery. A single mother and the writer Michelle Marie Warner explains what it means beautifully in a blog on the site PS I Love You. Warner writes, "Detachment with love means we let go of expectations and refocus attention toward ourselves. We don't try to control or manipulate outcomes. We allow others to be in charge of their lives, and we take charge of ours." This concept has been the hardest for me to practice not only with Jonah and Jacob but also everyone I care for in my life. Still, I know it is the most important.

It is worth acknowledging that there are many approaches to parenting, and we do not have to agree with each other's approaches all the time. Notice when you get into judgment around a parent's level and degree of control and use it as an opportunity to reflect on your own approach to parenting.

Taking care of our own lives? Letting go of control? Is this even possible? I think we need a big breath after reading all that. Or at least I do.

BREATH BREAK

Inhale, pause, exhale, pause, repeat.

Whether we choose to practice these less-attached approaches to parenting or not, reflecting on how we honor our children's autonomy can prepare us for the much bigger letting go's that we all inevitably face. Like, my letting Jonah have free rein of the playground was really preparation for his first day of pre-school, just as that first day of preschool will be preparation for his first time at summer camp or his first school dance or his first apartment. Or his wedding. And then I will have to do it all over again with Jacob? Excuse me while I am a puddle of tears

....

PARENTING IN PRACTICE
Janice's Story

For many yoga-practitioner parents, their practice is a sacred time. A time to disconnect from the distractions of the external world (ahem, their children) and devote solely to oneself. But Janice is at a very different stage. One where her children are grown and have families of their own. One where every phone call has become precious, even if it happens during asana practice, and even if she is simply picking up to tell her kids, "I'm doing yoga right now and can't talk."

Janice came to yoga somewhat later in life. She was fifty-nine and already a grandmother. She started practicing because she was facing her own mother's imminent passing and doing yoga helped her to disconnect both from her duties as a daughter and the responsibilities as the matriarch of her family.

Now over ten years later, things are quite different. Not only did Janice have to let go of her mom, sister, and a dear friend in the past decade, but as her grandchildren have gotten older, she has also observed that her role has shifted from mom the adviser to "Nannie" the support system.

The theme of the last ten years seemed to be letting go. The theme of her entire parenting journey has been letting go.

Where once her children needed her constantly, she has been feeling less and less needed. Where once she was her children's entire world, they now have entire worlds of their own. Where once she was the matriarch of her family, at seventy years old, she is starting to understand what her mother once said to her about feeling "put out to pasture."

Janice often says that "motherhood has many chapters." She has experienced the coming together and growing apart between herself and her children many times over in the past forty-five years, but even though she knows that any periods of space are for the best (as these are often periods when her kids are forging new heights in their own lives), she can still get thrown by those periods of disconnection.

Janice's daily asana practice helps her during those phases of separation and growth, and though it may only provide momentarily relief some days, as she says, "momentarily is better than nothing." Asana helps her because it is a tangible reminder of the very natural pattern of coming together and letting go that we all face in most aspects of our lives—from our relationship to our children to our relationship with our own bodies.

Just because her son may not call her every day for child-rearing advice and she and her daughter sometimes go through periods of space (although they are perhaps the closest they have ever been these days as her daughter just welcomed a third child), Janice knows that parenthood is not just those moments. In parenthood, love is the thread that keeps you connected to your children in even the most distant of times. It is the theme tying the most seemingly disparate chapters together.

So now, whenever the phone dings or rings, regardless of what she is doing, especially during yoga, Janice always tries to answer. The phone calls are so much more precious now, and though there are some periods when they seem to happen less frequently and others with more abundance, her practice reminds her that this is the flow of parenthood.

This is the flow of life.

....

LETTING GO OF OURSELVES

People seem to regularly talk about all the letting go we have to do with our children. There are even terms for it, like "empty nester," but what of the continual letting go we must do of the phases of ourselves?

From letting go of who we were before being parents, to our (somewhat) regained freedom when our children reach school-age and are more independent, to when children may move out of our home to build their own lives. Just as there are many chapters of parenthood, it helps to remember that parenthood is just a small book within the larger book of *our* entire lives.

This is really the essence of what our yoga practice is teaching us: this life is just a small chapter in the bigger book of our many lives and, ultimately, the one writing the book is our true Self.

This is the ultimate vairagya. Patañjali calls it *Para vairagya*: nonattachment to the small self.

Dr. Tigunait describes in *The Secret of the Yoga Sutra: Samadhi Pada,* "Para vairagya is the highest form of non-attachment, a state of consciousness in which we are fully established in our core being. In this state, the mind is so clear and tranquil that we see ourselves without distortion. Our self-understanding is so firm and bright that there is no need to remind ourselves that we are Consciousness itself. We know—with absolute certainty—that we are pure Seer, the very power of seeing itself."

Yoga returns us to wholeness. It helps us recognize that no matter how many chapters we go through, how many roles we play, how many losses we face or joys we gain, there is a part of us that is unchanging and ever-present. That same thread of love that ties us to our children, no matter how far away they may be, is the same thread of love that ties all the versions of our human self back to our ultimate Self.

FROM MAT TO FAMILY

One of the most effective skills Janice, who is not only the matriarch of a large family but also a respected therapist, taught me and teaches other new parents is the act of taking a beat before jumping in to react.

By sitting back for a moment, we leave space for our children to figure things out themselves. Janice's favorite mantra is "They'll figure it out," and as the parent of two children now in their forties, she assures us that they always do, and if they don't right away, they will eventually.

This exercise will bring in a lot of the previous work we have done in that it requires stillness and presence. This is the practice of learning to observe our children without expectation.

We watch television and movies for entertainment, but there is nothing quite as entertaining as observing your family—when you can remain objective, that is.

For *twenty minutes* one day, become like a stealth anthropologist and simply sit and observe. Observe both what is happening in front of you and your internal urges to meddle or get involved. You may want to review the nervous system chapter, which encourages you to keep an eye on your heart rate and breath cadence.

If someone asks for your help or you need to intervene, take *five breaths* before deciding how to respond. Use your judgment. Obviously, if there is danger, you must be ready to jump in more quickly, but try to see how your child is handling the danger first before you intervene.

Please note, if you have a newborn, not intervening for this length of time may not be feasible, so just try it in smaller increments. I love letting Jacob lie on his mat and seeing where his attention travels to.

But if your school-age child is getting frustrated finishing their math homework and you wait to swoop in, not only will you be better prepared to handle their distress, as you will have taken a few breaths and potentially calmed your own nervous system, but they may also figure it out first.

Or if your teenager starts telling you a story, taking five breaths before jumping in to offer advice may allow them to tell you that they came to their own conclusion. Through your sitting back, you may realize that they just wanted an ear to listen.

This exercise can be particularly effective during transitional periods when your child(ren) is/are becoming more autonomous. It will allow you to simply observe this beautiful life that you have created, without expectation.

Even if only for twenty minutes one day.

Ten Takeaways for Busy Parents

· All parents will face some form of letting go, over and over again, throughout their child's life.

- Patañjali's Yoga Sutra introduces us to the concepts of *abhyasa* and *vairagya*. *Abhyasa* means "practice" or "effort" and *vairagya* means "nonattachment."
- The practice of vairagya is endemic to parenthood. Letting go is the heart of the whole practice of parenting.
- The author and speaker Byron Katie often says that nonattachment is the key to loving unconditionally.
- There are entire systems of child-rearing that focus on nonattachment and giving the power to the child, such as Magda Gerber's RIE method of parenting.
- Many researchers have found these less-intrusive parenting styles to be incredibly effective in hunter-gatherer cultures.
- Just because we let go of our attachment to results or our children being a certain way does not mean we are abandoning them. The Al-Anon program for friends and family of alcoholics gives us the powerful phrase "detaching with love," which means we can continue to love those around us deeply yet let go of the need to control them.
- Parents will experience many chapters of coming together and moving apart throughout their child's lives.
- Oftentimes, the periods of separation correspond with times in a child's life when they are forging new paths or entering new important stages.
- Become a stealth anthropologist and try to observe your family without intervening at different times throughout the day. What do your children learn when given the space to figure things out on their own? What do you learn?

PART THREE

Connection

8

Living in Harmony

The most profound thing we can offer our
children is our own healing.

—Anne Lamott

.....

Sukhasana (Comfortable Cross-Legged Seat) with Sama Vritti Pranayama (Even Breath)

Each of us is beautifully unique in our own way. No two people
will ever look the exact same in any pose, just as no parent-child
relationship will ever be the same, even in a household with
multiple children; even amid multiples who are born within
seconds or minutes. Remembering to make the poses work
for each of us and our body on the mat can remind us to make
parenting lessons work for us and our family off it as well. But
first, we must get to know ourselves intimately to get to know
our unique needs.

Getting quiet and focusing on establishing an evenness of
breath and/or body is a great equalizer. It is an activity that all

of us can do, whether we are sitting on the floor or in a chair. Parenting is a great equalizer as well. It may not look the same home to home, but we can all set a similar intention of establishing connection and love.

Be kind with yourself if the breathwork portion of this posture is challenging. Taking care of others starts with taking care of yourself.

Sit on the floor.

Cross your shins and align your ankles beneath your knees for *Sukhasana* (Simple Cross-Legged Seat). If your knees are higher than your hips, consider elevating your sit bones with more blankets or a bolster. You can also prop up your outer knees with rolled blankets or blocks. Be comfortable.

Rest the back of your hands on your top thighs with your palms facing up.

If it feels safe, close your eyes or simply soften your gaze to the floor in front of you.

Once settled, begin Sama Vritti Pranayama. This means "even turning" or "even breath." It is also sometimes called "box breathing."

Inhale for a count of four. Pause and hold the breath for four (if you're able! See below for ways to modify). Exhale for four and pause at the base, holding for four.

That is one complete round. Repeat for five full rounds or as often as needed.

If the counts are too fast or too slow, choose a count that works for you, simply ensuring the breaths and holds are the same length.

.....

FINDING BALANCE IN OPPOSITES

When I think back to my teen years and early twenties, it boggles my mind that I was able to maintain the lifestyle I did. I moved fast, stayed up late, worked a high-intensity job in the film industry, lived on caffeine and cigarettes, and partied a lot. I was young and didn't have kids. I was still a kid myself in a lot of ways, but when I got an ulcer, I knew it was time to make some adjustments. Or more accurately, my older sister told me I needed to.

Late one night, in a steamy room in Santa Monica, my sister, Jennifer, took me to my first power yoga class. I had done asana many times up to that point, but it was mostly on video at home or in gym settings. I had never done fast-paced and strong yoga like this. Sweat was pouring out of me from my first Downward-Facing Dog, and even though it was ten at night when class got out, I was buzzing. It was the best I had felt in years, and after just a few weeks of attending classes almost every day, I quickly became aware of the discordances between my old life and my desired new one.

Naturally, as someone with an addictive personality, I overcorrected at first. Rather than going out drinking five nights a week and chain-smoking all day, I discovered Ashtanga yoga and centered my entire life around it to the point that I had no room for anything or anyone else. Instead of living off microwaveable meals, I became so austere about my food choices that I decided I should be vegan and gluten free (even though I've never been diagnosed with a gluten intolerance). Also, it is worth noting that I am naturally anemic; multiple providers have begged me to eat meat. Not to mention that I was still actively bulimic during this period, so despite my strict "healthy" diet Monday to Friday, when Saturday or Sunday would roll around, I continued to binge and purge, which many times included over-exercising like doubling up on superstrong movement classes.

I managed to get away with this "healthy" lifestyle for years, but as I began assisting and eventually leading teacher train-ings, I started educating myself more deeply on the study of Ayurveda and I realized that just because my choices appeared good on paper or worked for others did not mean they were the right choices for me or my body. The clearest indicators that things were amiss were my high anxiety, insomnia, ex-traordinarily dry skin and hair, my quick-to-anger impulses (particularly on Los Angeles's freeways), and my absentmind-edness and lightning speed, which led to multiple car accidents on those same aforementioned freeways. It also included my constantly upset tummy and hypersensitivity to everything around me. Oh, and let's not forget to mention the fact that I hadn't had a menstrual cycle in years.

As I sat in a lecture on Ayurveda one training, the master teacher listed off these very traits. She said that people who experience this are likely "*vata* types" and that when these traits were active, it was actually an indicator that the person was off-balance. She spoke of the fact that many of us are at-tracted to the very things that send us off-balance (hence my love for Ashtanga yoga and caffeine), but that in the Ayurveda system, opposites are what heal.

Over time, with the help of friends who intensively study Ayurveda and many, many books on the matter, I started to course correct. I adjusted my eating, adding in way more fats and oils and reintroducing meat. (Please note, I'm not advocating that you eat similarly. These were just the changes *I* needed to make at that point in time. I'm not a registered dietitian, and in fact, a major point of this chapter is about discovering what things work best for you, individually.) I adjusted my asana, favoring a much more grounded and slower pace to my obsessive and austere Ashtanga yoga habit. I started to let in a little more pleasure, including dating.

Fatefully, my menstrual cycle returned right before I met my husband (like literally weeks before), and as you now know, I was able to get pregnant and give birth to two healthy boys. I am no expert in the subject of Ayurveda, but once I was able to identify my constitutional nature and the constitutional nature of everything around me, I was able to make informed choices that have helped me find the balance I have been seeking my entire life.

WHAT IS AYURVEDA?

Let me begin by saying that Ayurveda is an incredibly rich and extensive subject that people dedicate their entire lives to following and understanding. We will barely scrape the surface's surface here in this chapter, but my hope in sharing this information is to give you yet another lens through which you may come to understand yourself more deeply. Then, if it resonates with you, you can take a deeper dive with the phenomenal experts and suggested resources provided at the end of the book. Or if you're a "dabbler" like me, you can use this abridged preview as an additional tool in your self-care tool kit.

Ayurveda is one of the oldest continuously practiced forms of medicine on the planet. The word itself literally translates to "the science of life," with *ayur* meaning "life" and *veda* meaning "knowledge" or "science." Ayurveda is not just about treating and preventing illness; it's a way of living. The art of being, as many practitioners say. It has been described as "one of the greatest and most complete systems of self-care ever developed" by the teacher and author Rod Stryker.

Ayurveda originated in the Indus Valley civilization as an oral tradition and was later put into text. It was not only practiced in India but neighboring countries as well, including Tibet, Nepal, and China, and is thought to be the basis of many other forms of traditional medicine. When India was colonized around the middle of the eighteenth century, Western medicine was pushed as normative and Ayurvedic practitioners were forced to move underground. It had a resurgence after India gained its independence in the early part of the twentieth century and is now practiced and respected worldwide.

One of the keystones to this holistic system is seeing people as whole beings within the greater macrocosm of their environment. It exemplifies how to bring our yoga practice off the mat by considering the health of individuals to not only be about the state of their physical body but also the state of their entire lives.

How will this help with our parenting? When we feel our best, we parent our best.

Something as simple as paying attention to when you should stop consuming caffeine during the daytime so you don't disrupt your sleep can have a tremendous effect on your overall well-being and thus your relationship with your kids. You don't just have to take my word for this either. There are an increasing number of well-designed clinical studies supporting what Ayurvedic doctors have known for thousands of years.

Ayurveda offers accessible daily tools for taking care of

ourselves, and as I have said in almost every chapter so far, we parents must fill our own tanks first in order to have anything to give our families.

Ayurveda believes that the fuel for those tanks comes from the three pillars of health: nourishment, restorative sleep, and a judicious use of our energy.

Before we look at the three pillars and how Ayurveda can help our parenting, we need to take a bit of a deeper dive in order to understand the general thinking behind this ancient school of medicine. As with any of the lessons we have explored so far in the book, just take what you like and leave the rest.

EVERYTHING IS NATURE

According to the original teachers of Ayurveda, everything in nature is composed of five elements. So, we'll start with a little element-ary school lesson. Get it? #momjoke. It is worth mentioning that although many Ayurvedic practices are supported by scientific research, anyone who's seen the periodic table knows there are more than five elements, but you can think of these as more philosophical than literal. They're also important for understanding and quantifying the attributes of nature as organized in Ayurvedic thought.

The Five Elements of Matter
(from Subtlest to Least Subtle)

- Ether (or space): Quality of, well, space; think of the sky
- Air: Quality of movement; think of the wind
- Fire: Quality of transformation; think of the sun
- Water: Quality of emotions; think of a river
- Earth: Quality of stability and rootedness; think of soil

Everything, from the areas that we live in, to the food we eat, to our pets, to we ourselves, is made up of some combination of these elements. In her book *Happy Healthy Sexy: Ayurveda Wisdom for Modern Women*, Katie Silcox explains, "Your elemental nature is a wild and wonderful 'fingerprint' that is unique to you."

Since everything is made up of these same five things, it not only means that we humans are all deeply interconnected but also that what happens in nature happens to us.

Have you ever noticed that people often seem to be in the same mood on certain days? Like how everyone in yoga class is half-asleep and lying on the floor in Savasana on rainy days, but that very same class time feels abuzz and extra chatty on a hot, spring day. Or how all the children in the neighborhood seem feral and wild on summer days, but in winter, the streets feel empty? There's a reason why it feels so good to have warm, hearty stew when it's cold out and fresh apricots when it's warm. We are nature and nature is us.

DOSHAS

While there are definitely days when everyone seems to be feeling the same thing, there are many more days where people have unique needs. Though all five of these elements are thought to be present inside all of us and everything, everything and everyone has their own unique formula. Our own unique formula of elements comes together to determine our *dosha*, our constitutional makeup, which is generally a blend of one or two of the elements, with trace bits of the rest.

Vata

ELEMENTS	Air and ether.
MAIN QUALITIES	Creativity and movement.
PHYSICAL EXPRESSION	Smaller boned and thin frame.
GENERAL VATA TRAITS	Sensitivity, including one's nervous system (prone to anxiety) and digestive system (prone to gastrointestinal issues).
VATA PARENTS WHEN OUT OF BALANCE	Spaciness and forgetfulness. An ability to learn quickly, but not having great retention. For example, vata parents may easily remember every single teacher's name and subject at Back to School Night, but forget once back home. They may miss deadlines when it comes to signing papers or appear scattered. Think "parent brain."
VATA PARENTS WHEN IN BALANCE	Creative, spontaneous, fast-moving, and fast thinking, making them great at imaginative play.
VATA ON THE MAT	Though vata types are generally attracted to flow and movement, this may bring them out of balance. Poses that can help balance vata are those that are grounding, like seated forward folds.

Pitta

ELEMENTS	Fire and water.
MAIN QUALITY	Transformation.
PHYSICAL EXPRESSION	Muscular build and medium-framed.
GENERAL PITTA TRAITS	Associated with a lot of heat, as such, pitta types tend toward having rashes, inflammation, or acne.
PITTA PARENTS WHEN OUT OF BALANCE	Tendency toward intensity and perfectionism, which may lead pitta parents to be quite critical and/or place a lot of pressure on their children. Tendency toward explosivity.
PITTA PARENTS WHEN IN BALANCE	Incredibly motivated and enterprising. A love of challenge and taking command, making them the CEOs of their families.
PITTA ON THE MAT	Tendency to be attracted to more heated practices, but these may create an imbalance. Balance pitta with poses that are more calming or symmetrical and poses that open the solar plexus and small intestines, which is where pitta is believed to accumulate. Think *Ustrasana* (Camel Pose) or *Setu Bandha Sarvangasana* (Supported Bridge Pose) on a block.

Kapha

ELEMENTS	Water and earth.
MAIN QUALITIES	Stability and heaviness.
PHYSICAL EXPRESSION	Larger-boned and hardy, including strong hair, teeth, and nails.
GENERAL KAPHA TRAITS	Savoring things, which may also lead to clinging and stubbornness.
KAPHA PARENTS WHEN OUT OF BALANCE	Kapha types may have difficulty or even devastation with big changes. For example, they may be more likely to experience an extreme loss of identity when the kids move out.
KAPHA PARENTS WHEN IN BALANCE	Great homemakers, cooks, and hosts.
KAPHA ON THE MAT	Kapha types tend to be attracted to slower-moving practices, but these may lead to an imbalance. Poses that help balance kapha are those that open the chest and stomach, where kapha is believed to accumulate. Movement-based sequences, such as sun salutations, are also beneficial.

If you would like to get an idea of which dosha you are, there are a lot of quizzes you can take online, or head to the Resources section for some suggestions.

BREATH BREAK

All right, now that we have this lexicon, we can get to know ourselves even more deeply, but first let's take a big breath. Inhale, pause, exhale, release.

....

PARENTING IN PRACTICE
Nikki's Story

In 2009, Nikki was at emotional rock bottom. Over the course of a year, her mother passed away after a long battle with cancer, her family lost their home due to the housing crisis, and all while caring for two young children, the youngest of whom would still wake frequently throughout the night.

Nikki was completely depleted. Her strong asana practice, which was once energizing, now only seemed to tire her further, and even when the new baby was sleeping (which was rare), she was wired awake, lost in anxious thoughts about her family's future and swimming in a sea of grief about her mother. If she did manage to fall asleep, she felt as though she could never reach deep sleep, toggling on the surface of wakefulness, ready for the next crisis.

Nikki was desperate for a change, but she didn't know where to begin. She barely had time to shower or eat full meals, often just eating the remnants of her toddler's lunch instead of fixing her own. Then she attended a talk on Ayurveda.

The part of that workshop that stuck out most for her was

learning about the three pillars of health: the foods we eat, restorative sleep, and a judicious use of our energy. Learning these, something clicked. She realized that she had been spread so thin and squeezed so tight, she truly had nothing left to give.

After attending the talk, she sought out an Ayurvedic doctor, but not without hesitation. Even if insurance does cover some part of alternative medicine treatments, it is often minuscule. Still, Nikki knew that it was worth the investment—*she* was worth the investment.

Minutes into their first meeting, the doctor took one look at her and said, "You need to make yourself a priority."

The first thing they did was see how Nikki could carve out space for herself. In one case, this was literal, like moving her yoga practice out of the living room and into a studio. She had been doing it at home, wanting to be available to her family, but that ready access meant it was never really her time.

Another adjustment they made right away was to Nikki's food. According to the Ayurvedic belief system, food is medicine. Rather than eating last or while on the go, which had meant sustaining herself on a lot of cold or prepackaged food, Nikki started taking the time to cook food that was warm and nourishing. Not an easy commitment for a mother of two toddlers.

The Ayurvedic doctor also looked at Nikki's sleep schedule, encouraging her to set aside time for naps, and (gulp) they discussed setting up a sleep routine for the baby.

All of these adjustments felt selfish at first. She was riddled with guilt, but as time went on, Nikki finally began to understand that to take care of her family, she needed to take care of herself.

After years of feeling run down and perpetually out of sorts, Nikki's tanks began to refill. Her creativity was reignited, and the mood in the entire household shifted. There was joy and excitement again.

All because Nikki started taking care of herself.

....

THE THREE PILLARS OF HEALTH

We've all heard the adage that we need to fill our own tanks in order to have anything to give others. Well, thanks to Ayurveda, now we know exactly the three tanks that need to be filled: nourishment, sleep, and energy.

Pillar 1: Nourishment

In Ayurvedic medicine, everything begins in the gut. One of the first things most Ayurvedic doctors do when working with new patients is to adjust their food. According to Ayurveda, food has the power to heal us and energize us or deplete us and exhaust us.

Have you ever eaten a piece of fruit that was so alive, you felt more alert as a result? I remember drinking orange juice in Bali that was so fresh, I felt like I had just downed an entire cup of coffee. Or conversely, have you ever eaten food that left you feeling heavy and exhausted after? Me, every time someone sends me those gourmet popcorn tins as a gift for the holidays and I eat an entire section in one sitting.

Look, I am no registered dietitian nor a licensed Ayurvedic practitioner. Full disclosure, as a family, we eat frozen food multiple nights a week and I still use a microwave. But I also always try including something fresh and alive with each meal, be it sautéed vegetables or fruit. Please be realistic about what works for you and your family.

Kathryn Templeton is a highly accredited clinical psychologist, yoga therapist, and Ayurvedic practitioner based in Connecticut. She is also the mother of three. All of her children are close in age, with two of them only being eighteen months apart, so she recognizes firsthand the challenges of feeding an entire family while running around between after-school activities. One of the pieces of advice she offers her clients is that if they must eat fast food, they should try to pick foods that will be the most digestible. For example, she suggests getting something fresh and unprocessed (if possible!). This includes options such as grilled chicken, whole grain breads, and salads.

Curious how you can know whether something is easily digestible? The same way you know that your little one did not digest that pineapple you gave them last night. Look at your poop. (Side note: Did you ever think about poop so much before raising a child? Even as a dog owner, I had no idea it would take up *this* amount of my attention!) Ayurvedic practitioners love talking about poop because it is an indicator of health. They typically say that a healthy body evacuates once a day in the morning and the bowel movement is odorless and well-formed.

But back to food.

Templeton encourages parents to have lots of vegetables on hand at home to accompany any frozen or boxed meals. She especially recommends selecting seasonally appropriate foods. This means eating the fruits and veggies that grow during the current season and in your part of the world. Of course, when the only healthy food you have access to is imported, you just do your best. Any veggie is better than none.

Templeton also recommends people eat their biggest meal of the day at lunchtime, when our digestive abilities are thought to be their highest, keeping breakfast and dinner lighter.

Something interesting to note is that, in Ayurveda, nourishment is not limited to food. It is anything we consume and would need to digest—from the conversations we have to the websites we visit regularly to the television shows we choose to watch.

Pillar 2: Sleep

If you are a new parent, talking about sleep may seem a little laughable. Like, "Duh, Sarah, I would sleep if I could." But sometimes what is preventing us from sleeping well is not a crying baby at night. My eldest started sleeping through the night at six months old and I was still waking up at 3 a.m. and unable to get back into a deep sleep for an entire year after that, and I know a number of parents who experienced the exact same thing.

Sleep is when the body and mind digest and repair. If we do not sleep enough, the body does not have the time and space to heal itself and we may get sick. Have you ever pulled an all-nighter for work or school and felt mild cold symptoms the next day? Well, multiply that by six months or more for new parents. Like the lines on a tree ring, you can always tell how many kids someone has by the number of bags under their eyes!

Lack of sleep not only affects us and our own body; it also affects the rest of our family. No one pays more dearly for our poor sleep than them. We are often quicker to anger or drop the ball on tasks more often when exhausted. So, what can we do?

Remember that the overarching goal of Ayurvedic medicine

is to live in harmony with nature. Nature is our guide, which means instead of relying on our phones to know what time to wake up or go to sleep, we can look to the sun.

Templeton calls following the sun's lead "circadian medicine," explaining, "When the sun rises, so do the birds and so should we. And when the sun sets, that's when we should start to work toward our own sleep."

Something as simple as dimming the lights and choosing to read a book (ideally not on a tablet) before bed instead of watching television can profoundly affect that night's sleep. Instead, what do most of us do at night? Keep the lights on long after the sun sets and watch a Netflix true crime documentary on a flickering screen.

Also, sleep hygiene is not just a matter of what we do right before bed but what we do throughout the day. This means looking at the amount of caffeine we consume and what time we stop consuming it. It means looking at the foods that we eat and the people we interact with and even the content we take in from our screens.

Simply resting during the quieter times of day—rather than hopping on our phones and powering through work emails when our children nap—can help fill our sleep tank, too. And remember that everyone's needs are different. I can't drink caffeine past eight in the morning, lest I be up all night, while my brother, Josh, literally drinks coffee until he goes to bed, and he has a teenager *and* a toddler! Paying attention to the effects of these choices will help you figure out what is best for you. This is also where an Ayurvedic doctor can be extremely helpful if you get stuck or want to go deeper. Many excellent practitioners offer sliding scales.

SLEEP FOR PARENTS OF NEWBORNS

For parents of newborns, sleep can feel like a faraway dream. One of our main jobs those first few months is to help our little ones establish proper sleep cycles. This makes it even more important to use the sun to guide our internal clock. Baby sleep experts may not agree on all things, but almost all of them suggest opening the shades and bringing in the light during the day and closing the blinds and dimming or turning off the lights at night.

Templeton acknowledges the challenges of sleep for brand-new parents, but she also encourages newborn parents that restorative sleep is possible when babies are around six to nine months and more in tune with the natural rhythms of the day. Fingers crossed our youngest adjusts more quickly than that!

Pillar 3: Energy

We talk a lot about "energy" in yoga and the word can be somewhat confusing or esoteric. In Ayurveda, this means the vital life force that gets you through a day.

Our energy tanks are not bottomless. Anyone who has ever experienced burnout knows you can completely wipe yourself out. You may get away with running on fumes for a short (or even sometimes long) while, but eventually you will become completely depleted. This can manifest in many ways from illness to exhaustion to explosive anger.

The original Ayurvedic teachings quantified this pillar as "management of sexual energy," but modern practitioners have begun viewing it more broadly, explaining it as management of our vital energy.

This is so much more than sex. It is about making wise choices about whom and how we spend our time. It means looking at what we are saying yes and no to. Are we overextending ourselves and taking on too much? Review chapter 6!

It is also about looking at our thoughts. Our thoughts are powerful, and where they go our energy follows. Are we wasting our precious resources comparing and contrasting ourselves with other parents on social media? Are we replaying some silly blowup we had with our child last week? Or anxiously anticipating what will happen this week?

Imagine if we took that energy and focused it entirely on being present with ourselves and our families.

ON THE MAT

The energy pillar may be the most applicable on the mat. Notice when you are overdoing it in postures. Are you overworking physically? Or competing with others in the room? Are you ignoring your body's signals and taking every single pose offered when you really should be resting? My teacher, Annie Carpenter, often asks her students to pull back their physical effort and see what they notice. She inquires, "Can you sense that as your effort diminishes—even just 20 percent—that your sensitivity is heightened? Your sensitivity to overstretching or overworking in your body but also the bigger picture: What are you creating in this moment?"

PREVENTION AS MEDICINE

Implementing even just a few self-care practices can help keep our three tanks much fuller, but first we need to debunk a few myths about self-care.

Number one: the myth that parents who practice self-care are selfish.

Self-care is not selfish. It is self-preservation.

I repeat: Self-care is not selfish. It is self-preservation.

Next, there seems to be a myth that self-care needs to be a huge overt experience, like a spa day or weekend getaway. Not true. Self-care can, and should, be something we do a little bit of every day. In Ayurveda, these daily rituals are called *dinacharya* and many are often completed first thing in the morning, before the rest of your family is even awake.

Finally, there's the myth that self-care is one-size-fits-all. Nope. It's totally personal. What I need to refuel is very different from what you need.

For an in-depth list of doable Ayurvedic dinacharya suggestions, please refer to Kathryn Templeton's guide "Simple Self-Care Tips for Parents" in the Resources section.

And just remember: the better we take care of ourselves, the better we can take care of our children.

FROM MAT TO FAMILY

There are a few parts to this exercise. I recommend doing this one at the end of the day.

First, in your journal, write down the entire day's activities from waking to evening. You can write this as a list of bullet points or more like an essay. Whatever is easiest for you to understand.

Next, let's check the levels on each of our three tanks using the following three measures:

Nourishment Tank

- FULL: you ate well and feel sated.
- LOW: you may have had one good meal, but the rest of the day was somewhat of a wash.
- EMPTY: you have not sat down to eat anything yet and/or everything was cold and processed.

Sleep Tank

- FULL: you woke up with the birds, feeling refreshed.
- LOW: you woke up around 7 or 8 a.m., but crashed midday.
- EMPTY: you are perpetually exhausted.

Energy Tank

- FULL: your energy felt sustainable throughout the day with little to no help from caffeine.
- LOW: your energy started strong but dropped midday and needed some help from sugar or caffeine.
- EMPTY: three cups of coffee later and you're still exhausted.

Now, reflect: Are you surprised with your results or were they to be expected? What factors do you think influence your tank levels? Refer back to what dosha(s) you may be. What effect does that have on your choices and tendencies?

Finally, can you commit to shifting one thing per tank tomorrow that may help refuel you?

Reminder that if you want to go deeper, simply head to the Resources section for a list of books, renowned Ayurveda practitioners, and Ayurvedic courses, and don't miss Kathryn Templeton's "Simple Self-Care Tips for Parents."

Ten Takeaways for Busy Parents

- Ayurveda is one of the oldest continuously practiced forms of medicine on the planet.
- The word itself literally translates to "the science of life," with *ayur* meaning "life" and *veda* meaning "knowledge" or "science."
- Ayurveda is not just about treating and preventing illness; it's a way of living.
- Ayurveda exemplifies how to bring our yoga practice off the mat by considering the health of individuals to not only be about the state of their physical bodies but also the state of their entire lives.
- We are nature and nature is us.
- Your dosha is your constitutional makeup based on what Ayurvedic practitioners call the five elements of nature: ether, air, fire, water, and earth.
- The three main doshas are: vata, pitta, and kapha. One of those tends to be dominant, but we can be any combination, including having all three evenly present, which is called "tri-doshic."
- Many people tell parents that they must fill their own tanks in order to have anything to give. Ayurveda believes that the way we fill our tanks is through the three pillars of health: nourishment, sleep, and energy.
- Self-care practices do not have to be grand or overt. Self-care can include a number of tiny rituals performed each day. In the Ayurvedic system, this practice is called *dinacharya*.
- Self-care is not selfish, it is self-preservation.

9

The Sharenting Dilemma

Comparison is the thief of joy.
—Theodore Roosevelt

.....

Upavistha Konasana
(Wide-Angled Seated Forward Fold)

During class, I love to give a lot of options. I know that it may be overwhelming at times, especially if one has had a long day taking care of everyone else and just wants to be told what to do, but when embraced, choices can be empowering and, in some ways, a relief. They remind us that there is no one way to do anything—that we don't have to fit someone else's pre-prescribed mold—whether that be in parenting or yoga. *Upavistha Konasana* (Wide-Angled Seated Forward Fold) is a common pose where people tend to look around the room in class or at other bodies online and in pictures and evaluate their abilities. We can always draw inspiration from others, but the second we start comparing ourselves to someone else, we can actually rob ourselves of discovering what we need as individuals. Just because every other kid in the class has a cell phone already does not mean yours needs to, too. Just because other parents attend every single school event and gathering does not mean you need to, too.

What do *you* need?

While seated, take your legs apart into a wide V. If your groin (inner thighs) feels tight or your back is quite rounded, consider bending your knees.

On an inhale, reach your arms up and on the exhale, fold up and over your legs. There are many gradations to explore here, from keeping your knees bent and sitting upright fully and being propped on fingertips or blocks or a chair, or folding all the way down until your torso, and maybe even your chin, touches the floor, grabbing your outer feet. Wherever you land is perfect for *you*!

Reach your heart toward your chin and your chin toward your chest.

Hold for fifteen long breaths.

Come to sitting and use your hands to close your inner legs back together.

.....

I AM WORTHY

According to my phone, I spend an average of eight hours a day on social media (the irony of that entire statement is not lost on me, by the way). That's the same amount of time many people spend their days working full-time. I justify it by telling myself that it's for my "job," too. I'm an "influencer" for a variety of brands and companies, so much of what I create online is for income, but that's not all I'm doing on there. It's a bit more complicated than that.

First, I really enjoy making content. There is a highly creative side to it, whether it's filming funny videos for TikTok or writing essays on Instagram. These outlets feel akin to when I was a little girl and used to borrow my dad's giant camcorder to record my most recent play. Second, it's a way for me to stay connected with those I love most. With so many of my friends and family living apart, it enables me to remain in touch, and it's also a way for me to share my sons growing up. My besties and I may not speak very often on the phone, but they still get to see my boys almost every day. Last, there is an element of community for me. I find great solace in being able to band together with strangers facing similar issues. It helps me feel much less alone when I can share about going through things such as my miscarriage, my eating disorder, or postpartum anxiety.

While I love it and it is such a huge part of my life (one-third of it, according to my phone's stats on my usage), there is an incredibly dark side to social media for me. Periods when it has a chokehold on me. Periods when I get fixated on it, not unlike how I can fixate on food or anxious thoughts. Periods when I devote so much of my mental energy to thinking about what content I am going to create that I'm incapable of being present with my children.

My self-worth gets very tangled up in it all, too. If my "views" and "likes" are high, I feel high. This is not unsurprising given all the current research confirming that "likes" and "views" can create a dopamine hit to our brain that is similar to when one takes addictive drugs. But it also means that when my engagement is down, I feel very low. So low that I sometimes question myself as a writer, a creative, and frankly, someone worthy of love.

It is during these phases that I must remind myself—sometimes even force myself—to turn off my phone and get on my mat. My yoga practice reminds me that I am not the amount of likes or follows I get, just as I am not defined by the poses I can or cannot do that day. As I watch my body and attention change every day and every year, I get to see in real time how much these external measures fluctuate and change. But perhaps more importantly, my practice reminds me that deep inside of myself is a part of me that is unchanging, undefinable, and perfect. Poses will come and go, just as engagement goes up and down, but the mat reminds me that who I am at my core—who we all are—is indefinable and immeasurable because our truth is so much more magnificent than we could ever imagine.

THE KLESAS

Parenting is hard enough as it is. Layer in the outside pressures of society's ideas of what a "perfect parent" should look like and we have a recipe for suffering. Full disclosure: I have had my children repeat something amazing to "get the shot" for Instagram. I have been completely checked out at holiday gatherings and events because I was more swept up with the Instagram reels or TikToks that I was creating than being present with my family. I literally TikTok'ed my way through labor with my second! I have gone down many a rabbit hole of looking at parents' social media profiles, where everyone looks happy and fit and put together, and then comparing my life against theirs.

The profiles we see on social media are curated versions of people's lives; they are aspects that people choose to share, not the entire picture. Thankfully, there seems to be a movement of profiles and influencer parents being way more "real." For example, the comedian, actor, and author of the book *Idiot: Life Stories from the Creator of Help Helen Smash*, Laura Clery, shared very rawly about her postpartum depression after her second child. The Canadian body-positivity influencer Sarah Nicole Landry, a.k.a. @thebirdspapaya, openly talks about her ever-changing relationship with her body after birthing four children. I try very hard to be a part of this movement on my social channels, but as someone who participates in this world every day, I have to confess to you that even when I post videos of myself crying because I am overwhelmed and exhausted by motherhood or pictures "celebrating" the changes of my postpartum body, I am still picking the "best" ugly-truth picture.

In the second pada of Patañjali's Yoga Sutra, there is a concept known as the *klesas*, the obstacles on our path to Self-realization. The very first one, the one that guides all the others, is *avidya*, ignorance of our true Self. A friend recently posted a meme on Instagram (I know, I know) that said, "People who shine from within don't need a spotlight." Well, I would like to revise that to say: people who *know* they shine from within do not need a spotlight.

Because we all shine from within. Yoga reminds us of that. Just as the big bang created the universe, we too were created from similar light and magic. I mean, think about how babies are made and created. We are all miracles.

There are five klesas in total and each feeds into the next. The first, avidya, forgetting who we truly are, can be thought of as the umbrella for all the others. It is said to be the root of all suffering and the cause of each subsequent klesa.

The next is *asmita*, or ego. This is often explained as "I-am-ness." These are the labels we misidentify as our entire reality when, beneath them all, we are so much more. Labels such as "I am a mother, I am a woman, I am brunette, I am a writer." We grip to these things because we worry that, without them, we will be nothing, but labels can be quite limiting.

Yoga reminds us that it is beneath them, where we are everything.

What roles do you identify with? How would you answer the statement "I am___"? Do you ever glimpse the perfection and pure light that you are beneath these roles? Or do you see that light and perfection in your child?

The third klesa is *raga*, or attachment. This is sometimes explained as "I want . . . " It is when we grip to what we think reality should be. For example, attaching to a particular behavior of our child's, like getting attached to them being "good" kids or measuring our worth by "likes" on social media.

The fourth klesa, *dvesa*, is "I don't want . . . ", or aversion. For example, disliking certain behaviors of our child or avoiding discussions as a family because they make us uncomfortable.

What aspects of your life or of your child do you cling to? What aspects do you abhor and try to change? The conscious parenting expert Dr. Shefali Tsabary often encourages parents to accept their children in their "as is" state, meaning to maintain our own peace, we need to learn how to accept them in this very moment—the good, the bad, and the not so pretty. What could that look like in your household?

The fifth and final klesa, *abhinivesa*, is often explained as "clinging to bodily life." Some modern scholars suggest viewing this from a bit of a different lens, which is less about death as in our final breath and more about the idea of the death of particular phases of our lives. For example, the suffering we experience when becoming new parents and guiltily mourn the ease of the days we were once childless. Or the suffering we face when wishing our teenagers were still little and would be sweet and cuddly, versus their new phase of never being home or rarely talking when they are.

What phases and changes over your child's lifetime have you resisted? Which have you embraced? How have those experiences been different for you?

ON THE MAT

Can you identify the klesas of asmita (ego/I-am-ness), raga (attachment), dvesa (aversion), and abhinivesa (clinging to bodily life) the next time you are on the mat? Are there certain poses that you measure your worth by? Are there certain teachers that you get attached to practicing with or spots in the room you must practice in? Are there poses that you roll your eyes to when the teacher offers it? Or just avoid completely? Are there any poses that elicit fear? Does your physical practice change when you remind yourself that you are so much more than any pose or phase of your practice?

....

PARENTING IN PRACTICE
Briohny's Story

The world-renowned yoga teacher and social media star Briohny Smyth has been in the public eye her entire life. She grew up a popstar in Thailand. It was hard navigating the nonstop press and public opinion as a young girl, so when she got pregnant at the young age of twenty-one years old, she decided to move back to the United States, where she was born, in hopes of avoiding the gossip and judgments. While many pregnant people and new parents receive unwelcome suggestions from outsiders, Briohny's experience was amplified because it wasn't just her family or neighbors who had opinions—it was an entire country.

Briohny didn't stay out of the limelight too long. She started teaching yoga in her midtwenties and rose to celebrity status quickly. One of the catalysts that propelled her into a "yoga-lebrity" was a 2011 video "The Contortionist " created by the luxury fitness club Equinox. In it, Briohny flows through impressive shapes in her undergarments while her then-partner, Dice Iida-Klein, another popular Los Angeles-based teacher, slumbers in bed. It is sexy, vulnerable, and powerful all at once.

At the time, social media sites like Instagram and YouTube were only just gaining stride, yet the video was seen around the entire world. Today, it has nearly sixteen million views. After it went viral, Briohny and Dice were booked for years out to teach workshops and festivals as a couple. As exciting as it was at first, Briohny was quickly reminded that with outside opportunity and fame comes outside pressure. It was especially hard on her relationship with Dice.

Briohny reflects that while she did love Dice dearly then, their marriage and business partnership may have been more about keeping up the external facade of being the perfect couple. It was when she and Dice had their son, her second child, that Briohny was reminded of what it means to love unconditionally and to show up authentically. Her children were, and always will be, a source of pure joy.

Unfortunately, the split in her attention between her children, who are her number one priority, and her business left little time for Dice or even herself. The couple publicly divorced in 2016. The separation helped shine an even brighter light on Briohny's budding realization that many of her decisions up to that point had been based on the outward appearance of things rather than her internal truth and connection to Self.

Nowadays, when it comes to sharing her private life with the public, Briohny is very intentional. One catalyst that helped reroute the direction of her "brand" was a beach photoshoot that at the time felt empowering and celebratory as a mother of two, but left her then-preteen daughter uncomfortable. After that, Briohny started setting limits on what she was posting, favoring educational videos over excess skin and "likes."

She also keeps things very compartmentalized when it comes to how much of her family or personal life that she shares, though she is not against posting photos from their travels or the occasional birthday message. If anything, these days, she seems to have to be placing more limits on her kids' social media habits, setting boundaries on their usage, and acting as a mirror when they slip down rabbit holes of endless scrolling or gaming.

Briohny's antidote for her family's social media passion and temptation to look outward for happiness is to do as many things together off-line and out of the public eye as they can. To "seek joy, versus likes," as Briohny beautifully says.

SHARENTING

With so many families living apart, social media has been a powerful way to remain in touch and to share your children growing up, but not everyone's profiles limit the access of that person's posts to family and friends, what many sites refer to as "private setting." If you share anything under the public setting, then people you've never met have access to your children and life. There is even a newer word for this practice called "sharenting," which is when parents share photos and personal information about their children online.

My husband and I regularly butt heads on this issue. I have always freely shared about all aspects of my life both in person and online, so when our first was born, sharing about him felt natural. Ben feels very differently on the matter and much prefers privately sharing offline to family and friend group chats. In an effort to compromise, we first made a deal where I had to get approval by Ben before any post I made about Jonah, but that lasted only a few months. Sorry, Ben. I will try harder.

I do sometimes look at other parents who never show their kid's face and wonder if I have made a poor decision being so open with ours. The thing with sharenting is that it often occurs without the child's consent, since it starts at birth, and the stats are a bit overwhelming. A UK study published in 2016 found that parents post an average of fifteen hundred photos of their children before they have even turned five years old. While this continues to be the study most major sources cite, I have to imagine that the number will significantly increase by the time this book comes out. I feel like I took that many pictures of Jonah and Jacob just yesterday at the beach.

I don't have an answer for us here. I think this is an ongoing issue that will continue to evolve over time and that every family is different. You have to do what feels right for you and then perhaps in time, when your children have more autonomy and awareness, you can bring them into the decision-making process.

COMPARISON IS THE THIEF OF JOY

With the advent of social media, life is no longer about keeping up with the Joneses down the street. Now, it's about keeping up with the Browns in Chicago, the Robinsons in Vancouver, the Gamburds in Israel, and the Franks in London. We are constantly bombarded with information on how other parents raise their children, from families at our child's preschool to superstars like Beyoncé and Jay-Z. Every time we log on to social media apps and look at another person's content, our brain makes comparisons whether we are consciously aware of it or not. Though the evidence-based research is still fairly limited by social media's infancy, most studies indicate that overuse at any age, meaning whether it's us parents or our kids online, is linked to increased anxiety, stress, sleep issues, higher levels of depression, and lowered self-esteem.

At the same time, there are a lot of benefits to social media. The ability to find support or specialty groups when one lives in places with limited resources or simply has limited time is undeniable. I could not have breastfed Jonah for nearly two years were it not for the breastfeeding support group on Facebook. Truly.

In addition to meeting new people, social media allows us to connect with people from our past or remain connected to people who live far away. On a global scale, corrupt governments have been overthrown thanks to people mobilizing through social media. From 2010 to 2012, the wave of protests collectively known as the Arab Spring that swept across the Middle East is often largely accredited to social media.

When you follow the right people or news sources, you can find a flood of good news and inspirational stories. However, if you take a wrong turn, you can end up in some serious vitriol, cyberbullying, and misinformation. It's a razor's edge and one we must traverse carefully if we decide to participate. Or you could choose to stay off entirely, like my best friend, Julie, who is a schoolteacher and mom of two. But considering that a 2021 Pew Research survey found that 72 percent of Americans use social media, compared to the 5 percent who used it in 2005, or that the National Alliance of Mental Illness estimates that three billion people across the world currently use it, the likelihood of someone in your family using it at some point seems quite high, no?

As we discussed in chapter 8, how we approach anything that we consume—media, yoga postures, even nourishment—can mean the difference between medicine or poison. Check out the Resources section for a web link to the National Alliance of Mental Illness's article "How to Have a Healthy Relationship with Social Media." Like many things, it all comes down to *how* we are doing something versus *what* we are doing.

MODELING INTENTIONALITY

One could call Vytas Baskauskas a reluctant social media star. Vytas's yoga classes are often mat to mat as he regularly draws upward of hundreds of students. He has appeared on multiple television shows, including the reality show *Yoga Girls*, which aired briefly on Z-Living and whose premise is discord between a new wave of yoga teachers, who embrace social media and the influencer lifestyle, and more old-school traditional teachers. Vytas was meant to represent the bridge between these two worlds. But despite all of his outward successes and reach, he is actually extremely uncomfortable when it comes to self-promotion and the limelight. He much prefers person-to-person connections to photoshoots and leading teacher trainings to selling products.

As such, Vytas has always been very intentional about how much of his seven-year-old son, Asa, he shares on his social media channels. Despite his mixed feelings about the platform (or maybe because of them), Vytas views Instagram as a personal photo album, and his son is a significant part of his life. There is no denying that pictures of him and Asa garner many more "likes" than an insightful share about yoga philosophy, but where Vytas and his coparent, Jacqueline, drew a very hard line is that they made an agreement to never use Asa to market themselves.

When Asa expressed interest in participating in one of his father's projects and filming a series of family yoga classes, Vytas was hesitant, but honored. The prep for filming ended up being incredibly joyous. It reminded Vytas of the early days when Asa would roll around on a mat next to him during his home practice, but on the day of filming, it was clear that, like his dad, Asa was not comfortable in front of the cameras. It was a long day for the little guy, and though Vytas encouraged him to see it through, as follow-through is an important value in his family, he may now reconsider including Asa in those kinds of projects; or as Asa is getting older and understanding things much more, Vytas will really make sure he knows what he's getting himself into before they commit to something like that again.

After all, Vytas himself is still not entirely comfortable with his own fame. He knows the toll that social media can have when we start to mistake "likes" for our worth. There's no denying that, like his parents, Asa is photogenic. He is also curious about their worlds, but perhaps Vytas's intentionality around social media will help Asa grow up with healthy boundaries already in place.

THE "GOOD ENOUGH" PARENT
AND THE IMPERFECT CHILD

Thankfully, the research is clear. We do not have to be perfect or even great for our children. Parents simply need be "good enough."

The idea (and relief) of not having to be the perfect parent was first proposed by the pediatrician and psychoanalyst Dr. Donald Winnicott in his 1973 book *Playing and Reality*, which talked about the "good enough mother." The concept was expanded to "parent" in 1987 by the psychologist Bruno Bettelheim in his book *A Good Enough Parent: A Book on Child-Rearing*.

The "good enough" parent is the idea that not only should we as the parent allow our children to see us make mistakes but that we should also encourage children to do so. In fact, these experts propose that it is through mistakes that humans may learn and grow the most. Not through our successes. As Hunter Clarke-Fields sums up in *Raising Good Humans*,

"When we allow ourselves to be human, and model healing in our relationships, we model that for our kids. They *need* to see you mess up, make amends, and still value yourself—so they know how to do it themselves."

The perfect parent myth is not only unattainable but when we attempt to parent from this perspective, it may also cause more harm than good. Studies show that perfectionism in families can lead to increased stress and unhappiness both with the parent and the kids. A recent article in *The Atlantic* entitled "Perfectionism Can Become a Vicious Cycle in Families," by Gail Cornwall, explores the detrimental effect of perfectionism. Cornwall writes that people who perpetuate it in their homes and with their children tend to be "perpetually dissatisfied, creating a tense and controlling home environment." Cornwall also warns about the contagiousness of perfectionism. That despite the negative effects on one's own well-being as the child of a perfectionist, numerous studies show that when we are raised by one, we are at high risk of becoming one ourselves.

Even if your family adheres to the "good enough" style, society perpetuates the perfectionist family image in several ways, too. The college admissions process alone is enough to make one's stomach churn, with college advisers now being hired when kids are freshman in high school (it was junior year when I was growing up, which in the States is eleventh grade, the year before you graduate). There are even advisers being hired for children to get into kindergarten in some cities! The additional cost for these advisers also furthers the inequity divide, as they are often expensive, and parents now must shoulder the expense of working with these advisers for multiple years.

Children have been reduced to test scores and grades, and suddenly in an effort to be the "perfect" family, we fall into the role of homework and grade enforcer instead of our children's safe space. And because there is so much pressure on families to measure their success by their children's achievements, including how the school system is set up (but that's another book), more often than not, parents end up just stepping in and doing the work for their children, which can lead to poor self-drive or performance in the long run.

Parenting experts—such as Jessica Lahey, a teacher and the author of *The Gift of Failure: How the Best Parents Learn to Let Go So Their Children Can Succeed*, and the authors of *The Self-Driven Child: The Science and Sense of Giving Your Kids More Control Over Their Lives*, William Stixrud, PhD, and Ned Johnson—implore parents to stop perpetuating the perfection myth and to instead embrace life's struggles. Most importantly, they collectively believe we should allow our children to fail and to fail often. Strixrud and Johnson write, "In fact, when kids are constantly shielded from circumstances that make them anxious, it tends to make their anxiety worse."

It seems that our drive to make everything perfect from the time our kids wake up to the time they put their heads down is not only exhausting for us but also for them.

In a system that values meritocracy, perhaps we would be better off striving for a little mediocrity?

Besides, we don't need external validation, like test scores or views on social media, to know we're doing a good job as a parent. We simply need to look at our children.

FROM MAT TO FAMILY

You often hear parents and parenting experts say that children may not listen, but they watch what we do. Modeling may be our greatest teacher.

Observe yourself for an entire day and take note of how much time you spend on social media or your phone, both when you are with your children and when you are alone. I am saying "on the phone" for those of you who, like my husband, may not be specifically on social network but still spend time on sports websites or news outlets. A lot of smartphones offer ways to track your usage directly or you could go analog and use a pencil and pad.

At the end of the day, simply observe and reflect. Are you surprised by how much time you spent online? Did you miss anything crucial that day when you were on your phone? Were there any spaces you put your phone away, and how were those moments? Remember not to judge yourself or berate yourself. We're here to learn and adjust, and awareness is the first step.

Now, let's set a few boundaries around your phone and/or social media usage.

Could you put bookends on what hours of the day you will use these? I have tried (not very well, but I keep trying) to be on social media only between the hours of 8:30 a.m. to 7:30 p.m. Vytas deletes Instagram off his phone every night before bed and will only reupload the app when he has completed his day's work around 5 p.m. This gives him a small window in the evening to be on and prevents incessant scrolling.

The goal coach, motivational speaker, and mother of three

Jacki Carr recommends buying a physical alarm clock and not even having your phone in your bedroom, so you don't use it before or after certain hours. Carr advises parents on goal-setting: "When setting goals (and boundaries)—finding our style and cadence, it is important to create a commitment we can stick to. What works for another parent might not work for you and it's okay to trial run and experiment with different ways of finding your own unique boundaries with social media."

Another thing to look out for is if there are specific times during the day or when you are with your children when you can simply just put the phone away or leave it at home. For example, no devices at mealtime. Meals can be a sacred bonding time for families and phones may get in the way of that.

I also try not to be on my phone when I am out and about with Jonah and Jacob. I mean, definitely not while driving, but even when we are out on walks. Again, I will sometimes have to make a phone call or text my husband about something, but I try my best to not be on a bench composing my daily IG post when we are at the playground. (Notice the specificity of that? Yes, I messed up and did this yesterday. You live, you learn!)

As Carr reminded us earlier, your boundaries will look totally different from any other parents. They may be much stricter or much looser (see chapter 6 to review the boundary spectrum). Reflect on what is appropriate and attainable for you and your family. Carr suggests asking yourself the questions "How is this supporting my whole life? How is this making me a great parent, partner, and friend?" Set yourself up for success by making tiny changes over time.

Remember that our goal is to connect with our children as much as it is about being true to ourselves. There is no such thing as the perfect parent nor do we want to be. Instead, let's simply set the intention that the times we are together are that much richer.

Ten Takeaways for Busy Parents

- Social media has positives and negatives, and the choice to participate, as well as the level of participation, is entirely unique to your family.
- "Sharenting" is the modern practice of parents publicly posting pictures and information about their children, often before they are of an age to consent.
- In Patañjali's Yoga Sutra, there is a concept known as the *klesas*. These are the obstacles on our path to Self-realization.
- Each klesa feeds into the next. The first klesa is avidya, ignorance of our true Self, and is believed to be the root cause of all of our suffering.
- The additional four klesas are asmita (ego/I-am-ness), *raga* (attachment), *dvesa* (aversion), and *abhinivesa* (clinging to bodily life).
- The "good enough" parent is the idea that we should allow our children to see our mistakes as well as encourage our children to make mistakes, too.
- Many experts agree that it is through our mistakes and discords when we grow the most.
- Perfectionism parenting can lead to challenges both for the parent and the child enduring it.
- The greatest valuation of how our children are thriving will not come from social media "views" or test scores or college acceptance letters. The greatest measure of how our children are doing is them.

- Setting boundaries around social media and/or technology usage can help us carve out times during the day when we are simply with our children for the sake of joy versus "likes." In doing so, we may be able to connect to our deepest Self, too.

10

The End Is Also the Beginning

Your children are not your children.

They are the sons and daughters of Life's longing for itself.

They come through you but not from you,

And though they are with you yet they belong not to you.

You may give them your love but not your thoughts,

For they have their own thoughts.

You may house their bodies but not their souls,

For their souls dwell in the house of tomorrow, which
you cannot visit, not even in your dreams. You may
strive to be like them,

but seek not to make them like you.

For life goes not backward nor tarries with yesterday . . .

—Kahlil Gibran, "On Children," *The Prophet*

. . . . .

Savasana (Corpse Pose)

No pose teaches us about endings more intimately than *Savasana* (Corpse Pose). After all, the literal translation of the word *sava* is "corpse." In addition to resting your body and mind, some say the whole purpose is to get familiar with death. But just as it's a profound lesson in letting go, so too can it teach us to begin again. When we come out of it, we usually roll into a fetal position before coming to sit, representing a rebirth on the other side of our practice. We are not the same person after we come to the mat, just as we are not the same person after we have children. But like we talked about in chapter 5 on tapas, this rebirth is not about becoming someone or anything new. It is a return to who we truly are.

Come to lying on your back. Separate your feet slightly wider than your hips and have your arms a few inches from your sides.

Allow your legs to fall open. If your low back is sensitive, bend your knees with your feet on the floor or keep your legs straight and place a rolled blanket underneath your knees. If lying down is not comfortable for any reason, you are welcome to find a seated position that suits you instead.

If it feels safe, close your eyes or cover them with a towel or pillow.

Take a full breath in through your nose and exhale it out through your mouth with a big sigh, "Ahhh." Let your breath become automatic once again.

Rest here for anywhere from three to seven minutes.

When you are ready to reemerge, hug your knees into your chest and roll to a side, pausing in the fetal position.

Use your hand to press up to sitting and sit quietly for a few moments.

Before diving back into the flow of the day and life, assess how you feel, renewed and reborn.

.....

MY (LACK OF AN)
EDUCATION ON DEATH

I wouldn't say I was in denial of death, but considering my life choices in my teens and early twenties, one could say that it was far from something I was aware was a reality. My mother had worked hard to make sure that death didn't touch me when I was growing up. If we had to put a dog down (which we did many times over the years), she always seemed to show up with a brand-new puppy the same day.

"We had to put Cleo down. Meet Charlie," she would say in the same breath.

When Nana, my mom's mom, passed, there was no discussion. I don't even remember my mom crying, and when I was acting out that week (likely trying to process the profound realization that people die), I was punished for my behavior rather than anyone sitting down and explaining to me the family's theory of death or what happens after we're gone.

My first memory of being shrouded from death was when I was around three or four and I wasn't allowed to see Walt Disney's *Bambi* because the mama deer dies in the beginning. I'm not sure I've ever seen it to this day and still scroll past it quickly when Jonah and I are deciding which movie to watch some afternoons.

When I absolutely lost it on the car ride home after Barbara Hershey's character passes from cancer in the Bette Midler movie *Beaches*, my mom coldly reassured me, "I'm not going to die, Sarah," more annoyed than sympathetic, ominously ashing her cigarette out the window. I'm not even sure I ever developed my own theory of death, other than picturing Albert

Brooks's 1991 movie *Defending Your Life*, where the characters sit in a big theater in heaven and watch a movie of their lives while judges determine whether they should be sent to heaven or hell. Yes, I watched a lot of movies.

But then starting in 2008, when I was in my midtwenties, one close family member after another passed away. It started with my brother, who took his own life on his forty-first birthday. Followed by my great-grandmother and great-uncle, both of whom I was close to. Then my aunt—my mom's sister—and another great-aunt. But the death that transformed my worldview and changed every fiber of my being was when I lost my mother.

I had never experienced a loss like that before. She was my best friend, my confidant, my roommate. I lived with her for most of my life other than college and a sorry attempt at early adulthood, though I quickly moved back in upon her diagnosis of stage IV lung cancer.

She got to see me teach yoga once. Hair shorn from the chemotherapy and perched on a puffy chair in the corner of the Lululemon, Brentwood store. She had to lean forward on her cane to see better, which she was using because the metastasized tumor on her spinal cord was so enlarged, she no longer felt her feet. She cried at the end when I brought everyone through a final AUM; for a woman of English descent, tears were a rare sighting.

While in the early years of my life my mom tried to shield me from death (it is worth noting these also corresponded to her heaviest years of her drinking), when she finally faced her own death, she took a completely different approach. By the time she was diagnosed, she had been sober from alcohol for over a decade and extraordinarily dedicated to the program of Alcoholics Anonymous. So much so she was often called the "mayor" of her Saturday night meeting. In her last months, our home was a revolving door of sponsees paying homage at her bedside. But her sobriety had inspired another path

She had become steeped in Eastern philosophy and specifically Buddhism. In addition to devouring everything the Dalai Lama ever wrote and every translation of the Dhammapada she could find, she meditated daily. Even at the very end of her life, when she was gasping for air, she would close her eyes and connect to her true Self.

Her comfort around death inspired me to seek consoling texts of my own from the yogic perspective. One of the texts that was most pivotal for me was the poem the Bhagavad Gita, found within India's great epic *The Mahabharata*. There are many translations of this and I gobbled them all up. It was hearing Krishna educate Arjuna on reincarnation, especially the metaphor that this body we are in is just an article of clothing, that helped me feel reassured.

When my mom died, I was devastated, but the sting was lessened by my belief that we will be together again, just as we likely were many lifetimes ago. If we are not, then maybe she has achieved liberation, and how could I ever deny her that? And despite the fact that I miss her every single second of every single day and wish she could meet my sons, this way of viewing life—that death is not really the end but a new beginning—helps me get through the time I have left in this lifetime without her.

THE END IS OFTEN
ALSO THE BEGINNING

Parenthood is a menagerie of firsts and lasts, often interwoven together. The first time your child walks is the last time they will crawl. (Well, in theory. Jonah started playing "baby" and crawling again as we neared Jacob's due date.) The first time they sleep in their big bed is the last time they sleep in their crib. (Again, in theory! This could take a few years.) The first time they drive their own car may be the last time they need you to be their daily personal Uber. (Unless their car is in the shop, but you get what I mean.)

Someone once said to me, "We remember the first time we pick up our children, but will we remember the last?"

The end can be a challenging concept for many human beings, but it appears particularly hard for those of us in the West (Europe, Australia, Canada, and the United States), where we seem to do everything that we can to prevent and deny it, from excessive medical interventions to shrouding death away from the public's eyes in funeral homes and cemeteries. However, if we look to cultures that celebrate death, like Mexico with Día de los Muertos or, of course, India, where yoga originated, we may be able to learn some valuable lessons that can help us face this inevitable season of life.

Varanasi is often considered the most sacred city in all of India, perched near the opening of the Ganges River. This is where people from all over the country bring the bodies of their loved ones for cremation. Cremation is common amid many sects of Hinduism because the body is believed to be a temporary vessel, and when the ashes are thrown into the

Ganges River, it is believed that the soul has a better chance of attaining moksha, or liberation, and thus breaking the cycle of death and rebirth.

Varanasi is the only place in all of India where bodies are burned every day and all day. The reason so many people spend all their resources to bring their family member's bodies to this holiest of places is because it is believed to be the home of Lord Shiva. It is also the place where Gautama Buddha gave his first sermon.

The first time I traveled to Varanasi, India, I admit, I was afraid to see the "burning bodies." I naively assumed it would be grotesque and sad, but being there amid the hordes of people along the ghats and seeing the dots of boats with tiny flames for offerings, I understood that these death ceremonies are much more celebrations.

And the death ceremonies of Varanasi are not only beautiful. They are also often being completed right alongside everyday occurrences. Like, you will commonly see people bathing in the holy waters or children playing, just a few feet down from a burning body. This is another way that some cultures profoundly differ from one another when it comes to approaching death. Not only does death happen out in the open but it happens right alongside life.

Kelly Phillips Badal, a journalist for *Travel & Leisure* magazine, described it vividly in a 2015 article for the publication. Badal wrote, "And even though death is on Varanasi's center stage, life boils here. You may see teenagers snapping selfies with a dead relative burning upon a pile of sandalwood, chanting women washing their clothing at the bottom of a crowded ghat, or gangs of men shouting and slapping at cows to nudge them along as they shoulder a shroud-wrapped body on a bamboo litter, bumping you abruptly out of their way as they pass. The kaleidoscope of colors, sounds, and scenes will overwhelm you—and will stay with you, too."

The author of *Meditation with Intention: Quick & Easy Ways to Create Lasting Peace* and public speaker, Anusha Wijeyakumar, was born and raised in Sanatana dharma or Hinduism and has been immersed in yoga and Vedic philosophy her entire life. She observes that in the West, a lot of the lessons of yoga have been watered down, theorizing that this is "perhaps due to people placing an Abrahamic lens on many of the ancient Hindu and yogic teachings." Wijeyakumar points out that you can't only pick and choose parts of yoga philosophy that suit your views. And especially, you can't talk about karma, the law of cause and effect, and then ignore reincarnation, because "karma and reincarnation are deeply intertwined."

In her home, she is very open with her three-year-old son about death. When an animal dies in one of his beloved animal shows, she simply reminds him, "Death is a part of samsara, the cycle of birth, life, and death before we return to God." There is no effort to hide death or shield him from its pain because it is not seen as painful; it is a part of life. Being raised in the Vedic and yoga traditions, she views death not as an end but a beginning of another of the millions of lives beings have, or complete liberation for some with the ultimate goal of samadhi, union with God.

In his book *Light on Life*, B. K. S. Iyengar shares that he did not cry though his wife died suddenly and unexpectedly. He writes, "I did not cry at her funeral. My soul loved her soul. This is love. It's transcendental and transcends the separation of death. If my ego, my small self, had been the source of my feelings for her, then I would have cried, and mostly I would have been crying for myself."

BREATH BREAK

If you want to learn about the cyclical nature of life, simply observe your breath. Inhale, pause, exhale, pause, repeat.

THE MANY INCARNATIONS OF PARENTHOOD

Reincarnation does not only happen across lifetimes. We also live many lives even in this one. We especially live many lives across the journey of parenthood. To be a parent is to grieve a thousand deaths.

But when does one become a parent? Is it when you bring a child home? Or when you see those two lines on the stick? What about parents who foster or adopt? What about parents facing infertility and subsequent losses?

It is my belief that parenthood begins the moment you set the intention to have children. Sara Hess and Matt Champoux are both yoga teachers based in San Francisco. They have been together for seven years and tried to get pregnant for two of those. In 2018, Sara was diagnosed with stage IV endometriosis. After a surgery removing the endometriosis, the doctors told her she had an extremely low ovarian reserve and likely, infertility. For those with infertility, every month one gets their period or sees a negative pregnancy test result can feel like a funeral, even if there is no physical loss.

Sara's fertility experience took her on a "hero's journey," as she calls it. It tested her and her husband Matt's inner resilience, their relationship, and their desire to be parents, all of which thankfully only seemed to strengthen each month. Her yoga practice became an inner sanctuary and safe place for her to process, heal, and listen. Her mat would meet her exactly as she needed to be every day, whether that was angry, sad, hopeful, or at peace. But the biggest takeaway from this experience was learning how to take care of herself and to be truly "full."

Prior to trying to conceive, Sara put all her energy into her yoga asana practice and teaching career, leaving very little for herself and ignoring important cues from her body. While outwardly her career was thriving and she appeared fit and healthy, inside she was running on empty. When she started trying to get pregnant, Sara refocused her efforts on self-care and learning to listen to her body. She worked hard to redirect the precious energy she once poured into the grind of it all, back into herself and her family. Even before a baby arrived, Sara understood the important lesson that parents must take care of themselves first to have anything to give their children.

Important update (and potential trigger warning): Since I wrote this, Sara and Matt have just recently given birth to their first child. I only share this because it is their path and truth. I acknowledge that this is not the path for many who are trying to conceive.

I suffered a miscarriage before my first son. My sister-in-law suffered six before my second niece. One in four pregnancies ends in miscarriage and apparently, it's one in three if you get pregnant after thirty-five years old. The moment that desire to bring a little one into your life is sparked, the reality of loss is sparked right alongside it. With both pregnancies, it seemed like the second those two lines appeared on that pink stick, I started worrying about both the potential loss of the new baby and the loss of my current life. No one tells you this part when you are first deciding to have children, but parenthood = grief.

And not just grief around losing the child or them growing into new phases. Grief around who you once were, too.

If you carry a child in your body, there is often some grief around the body that once was. Sure, many of us embrace the burgeoning belly, knowing there is a beautiful purpose to this growth and that it is temporary, but there is still a loss. A loss of agency and a loss of choice. When I got pregnant with our second, as joyful as it was, it was very challenging to not be able to keep up with my toddler. Or eat deli meat. I know, I know, but, personally, I think this view of the mother as the ultimate martyr who sacrifices everything for their child is unhealthy and outdated. For the sake of our mental health and living authentically, it is important to acknowledge the griefs just as much as we do the joys.

And that's just pregnancy. No one really prepares you for the "complete shit show" that is newborn life (direct quote from my brother, Geoff). People throw baby showers and gender reveals and celebrate the incredible love coming your way, but no one sits you down and explains, "Though you will be the most in love you have ever been, you may not be able to shower for a few months and you will miss your freedom at first."

As much as we grieve our autonomy when our children are newborns, they grow rather quickly and our grief changes from missing our independence to missing the feeling of their little body constantly on our chest. You mourn the pitter-patter of their feet down the hallway when learning to walk, as they start running around the neighborhood and riding their bikes.

Or you grieve the interminable stories they told as school-age children, when suddenly they become silent, brooding teens who only appear in the kitchen for fifteen minutes a day to make food. The grief grows in different ways, just as they do.

As our children change, we are asked to change, too. Watching our children grow up asks us to embrace the cycle of life and death over and over again while also letting go of resistance around those changes. How many times have you felt the urge to dig your fingernails into the moment and attempt to keep everything in a time capsule? Thankfully, in addition to yoga being an ultimate guide to helping us embrace the changing seasons across our life and lifetimes, we also have another incredible guide: nature.

....

PARENTING IN PRACTICE
Tamika's Story

Though Tamika and her wife, Lenie, only started their urban farm and inclusive outdoor wellness center, the Ranch Houston, in 2020, Tamika has borne witness to countless changing seasons across her lifetime. She has experienced these major endings and beginnings with her personal relationships, her body, and on her yoga mat. But it has been owning a farm and living amid the elements and ever-evolving harvests that has helped Tamika really appreciate the indelible truth that change is simply the nature of life.

One of the first and perhaps most profound periods of transformation Tamika experienced was at twenty-one years old, trying to balance having a newborn while also completing her undergraduate studies at the University of Texas. At first,

Tamika was committed to not letting being a new mom deter her studies, but after a while, the pressure was insurmountable. Despite powering through study sessions with a crying baby across her lap, Tamika ended up skipping out on her final exams that winter. In hindsight, she believes that she may have been suffering from undiagnosed postpartum depression. It was clear she needed a break, but that didn't mean she needed to give up. Much like she now encourages students in her yoga classes, you don't always need to come out of the pose entirely; just back off a bit.

After a year and a half of focusing on her new child and healing her body, Tamika returned to the University of Texas ready to complete her studies. She graduated that summer with her mom and daughter, Joie, cheering from the stands. And she also cheered for herself as she had gracefully turned a seeming ending into an entirely new beginning.

When Joie was in kindergarten, they started to do yoga together. In addition to her natural resilience, Tamika feels that it is her yoga practice that has really helped support her through the continually changing seasons of her life. Watching her body and breath change day to day is a reminder of the impermanence of this life.

Embracing the inevitability of change on her yoga mat helped her deal with her mother's early onset Alzheimer's and eventual passing. It helped propel her out of corporate America, where she had started working after graduation and was feeling unfulfilled, and onto the path of education, eventually obtaining a master's degree and teaching Spanish language, history, and literature. Yoga was also the place she came to heal emotionally after being dismissed by doctors for years who blamed her weight for her chronic hip pain. And the mat was where she literally healed after finally receiving the hip replacement, which she strongly suspects could have been avoided had the doctors taken her seriously to begin with.

The hip injury and eventual surgery also taught Tamika how much our bodies can change in an instant, as she had to say goodbye to certain poses and ways of practicing. But closing the door on one approach to practice allowed another door to open. While she continues to teach and practice stronger-level vinyasa flow classes, after her surgery Tamika became deeply immersed in the style of yin yoga and is now one of the world's leading yin yoga trainers and master teachers.

Tamika's asana and meditation practices were also incredibly helpful when her daughter turned seventeen years old and began blossoming into her own woman. Things especially changed when Joie told her mom she wanted to have a baby at a young age rather than going to graduate school or focusing on a career path directly out of college. Though Tamika felt some resistance at first to her daughter's choice, her life and yoga practice reminded her to trust the ever-changing seasons coming their way. And Tamika and Lenie had begun the farm by that point, so they had borne witness to nature's changes right before their very eyes.

Tamika has experienced many unexpected beginnings, but none has been more beautiful than the recent arrival of her granddaughter. Amid the fields of fruit-bearing plants of the Ranch Houston, this very special welcoming place that she and her wife created, their granddaughter is truly the most incredible bounty of all.

HOW YOGA CAN TEACH
US TO EMBRACE DEATH

What if rather than avoiding it or denying it, we lived with death constantly at the forefront? Could that change how we live? My mother's dying and death transformed my view of the world, and though it was one of the hardest things I have ever gone through to date, it led me to have an infinite appreciation for every single moment. I finally understood that it is in befriending death that we can truly appreciate life.

It is also in embracing that we are merely temporary guests here in our body that we can embrace the truth that we own nothing in this world, least of all children. As the Sufi poet Rumi said, "This being human is a guest house." Well, this being a parent is, too.

Remembering that Jacob and Jonah are just here with me temporarily helps me get through the hardest of moments. I come back to my favorite mantra from chapter 3: "This is all temporary." Bleary-eyed and milk-covered at four in the morning with a newborn who has no intention of going to sleep, I utter the words "This is all temporary." Sitting on the floor of the grocery store while my toddler wails and kicks his legs, "Temporary." That feeling like my heart is being torn in two while one child cries for me in a different room, but I am stuck tending to the other, "Temporary." It does not mean I cannot grieve the life I once had or the way things once were. It simply means that I try to hold both truths at once. I miss sleep, and I know these long nights will pass. I miss easy shopping trips, and I know he will be grown and out of the house before I know it. My heart breaks when I can't focus on both kids at once, but I know (hope) they will one day be best friends for life.

Even (and especially) the most beautiful moments we share are all temporary. Now, acknowledging the temporality of it may not always diminish the challenge of certain periods. It can simply help at times to remember that this is all a privilege. Parenting is a privilege, and approaching life and parenthood from this lens has been hugely transformative for me.

Another way that embracing the temporality of parenthood helps is that it encourages us to maintain our own sense of identity, separate from our children and separate from being a parent. If we become completely enmeshed in our children's lives, we can lose our sense of who we truly are. Remembering that even the most important roles of our life are just that, roles, helps us both appreciate them and ultimately not attach to them.

Tamika Caston-Miller, the co-owner of the Ranch Houston whom we met earlier, was raised in a very traditional Southern Black Creole family, where there is a clear hierarchy of roles between the elders and the children. The children do what their parents tell them to do, and there is a sense of what Tamika identifies as "ownership." As she explains, "In my family, love looks a lot like obedience."

But Tamika's approach to her relationship with her daughter is very different from most of the generations before her. In her eyes, her daughter is not *hers*. She is in her care. As such, Tamika often refers to herself as her daughter's "steward," even though she gave birth to her.

This has not only helped Tamika appreciate the time they have together but it has also helped her maintain her own identity separate from being a parent. She credits her own mother with planting this seed that is helping to break generational patterns of viewing children as one's own, but it is also her yoga practice that has helped her feel most comfortable with the reality. On her mat, Tamika is reminded again and again of the temporality of nature and the impermanence of this life.

FROM MAT TO FAMILY

When we look to nature, we see that death is just part of the greater cycle of life. Every winter the leaves fall from the trees, but every spring, they return.

We are going to practice a visualization meditation, imagining nature's cycles, and then you will play with visualizing the natural cycles throughout your child's life. Depending on the age of your child or where you live in this world, this practice may require some *vikalpa*, imagination. Of course, if you get stuck or live in a climate that is sunny and warm year-round, like I used to in LA, you can always Google "changing seasons."

Come to a comfortable seat or lie on your back. If it feels safe, close your eyes, or find a soft gazing point. Take a few deep breaths in through your nose and out through your mouth. Simply observe your breath. An entire life cycle is present in a single breath—the initiation of our inhale, the sustainment of the pause, the destruction of the exhale, and the emptiness before beginning again.

Start to think of summer. What does summer look like where you live? What does it feel like? The warm sun upon your skin. The scent of sunscreen and chlorine. Can you picture the trees verdant and full? Or the browning grass? The sounds of the birds and the taste of a summer fruit?

Now, begin to imagine the transition toward fall. How do you know when the change is coming? Is it the cooler breeze or changing light? The shorter days and longer nights? Picture nature as it transitions, the leaves falling from the trees and the winds picking up. What are the sounds of fall? What is the taste of fall? Squashes and pumpkins and cinnamon.

What does the air feel like when it becomes winter? The assault of cool air against your cheeks. The barren trees and sound of crunching snow beneath your feet. The smell of some-one's fire. The feeling of warm soup or cider in your tummy. In the Northern Hemisphere, the glow of holiday lights warming up the midnight sky. How the darkest day of the year can be the brightest when we are with our family.

And now imagine the first sign of spring. Is it the budding leaves or flowers poking through? The return of the birds and the bugs? Feel the warmth of sunshine on your face while your arms may still be cool. The smell of fresh rain and flowers. The return of life. The taste of fresh salads and juice. Children on bicycles and neighbors waving "hello."

As spring shifts to summer, the days become longer and warmer. More time is spent outside and in the water. Those cool breezes become like warm blankets wrapped around you. And suddenly it is once again the brightest day of the year. But as much as we bathe in the sunlight and dance amid the cloudless sky, we remember that tomorrow, the days will get shorter, and this cycle will begin all over again.

Take a deep breath in and out. And now take a few moments to visualize the seasons of your child's life. If they have been with you since infancy, picture the shift from their warm little body on your chest to sitting upright on your hip. From lying down and being content with a hanging toy above to taking apart your kitchen and playing in a sea of pots and pans. From their chubby little cheeks and funny language to lengthening out and speaking more clearly. Picture the shift from when you had to walk them to the door of school to catching the bus for themselves.

Can you see them clearly as they transform from school age children doing their homework in the dining room, swinging their little legs under the chair, to getting into their own car? To wearing a mortarboard cap at their graduation? To waving goodbye at the airport as they leave for their first adult adventure?

Each child is unique, so please take your time. Picture the seasons you have already weathered together or imagine a future that has not yet happened. Take your time and feel into each shift, both the loss of the old phase and the gain of the new period.

Take a few more deep breaths. Slowly start to bring your awareness back to the present moment. The feel of the floor beneath you. Your breath in your chest. If your children are within earshot, listen for them. Maybe they're on your lap; feel them. If your eyes were closed, slowly open them and return to this moment.

Ten Takeaways for Busy Parents

- *Savasana* gives practitioners an opportunity to explore death and endings, but it also allows us to experience rebirth, as we often roll to the side in a fetal position and rise afterward.
- Many cultures view death not as something to be avoided or feared but a part of life and even something to be celebrated.
- Parenthood is a menagerie of firsts and lasts, often interwoven together.

- Reincarnation does not only happen across lifetimes. We live many lives even in this one.
- When does one become a parent? My belief is that the moment the desire to have a child is sparked, one begins their journey.
- Watching our children grow up asks us to embrace the cycle of life and death over and over again.
- We see the cycle of death and rebirth in nature. The ebb and flow of the moon and the waxing and waning of the tides.
- If we can remember our children are just here with us temporarily, it may help us get through the hardest of moments.
- Embracing the temporality of parenthood can help us maintain our own sense of identity, separate from our children and separate from being a parent.
- Being a parent is just one part of us, just as this lifetime is just one part of our many.

11

The Yoga of
Parenting Sequence

While each pose and each lesson we explored are important to highlight and explore individually, the reality is that in families, we cycle through multiple experiences, rhythms, and lessons within single days.

Sean Gray has owned a virtual yoga studio, ran yoga festivals, and raised two girls. He is also an avid surfer. Sean observes that much like yoga and parenting, parenting and surfing have a lot of similarities. He explains, "It takes presence to see with clarity what the wave is presenting to you, agility to be able to shift and navigate that moment, balance to avoid getting knocked off your center, courage to willingly ride into uncertainty, and surrender to embrace the unknown outcome that ultimately comes with each wave, knowing you've done your best. Just like each day as a parent."

By weaving together all the concepts and poses we have explored throughout this book into a single sequence, it gives us the opportunity to practice surfing the waves of parenting on our mat, so when those same challenges and waves come up off it, we can be more prepared (or at least a little more prepared).

Feel free to improvise by adding in transitions or additional poses that feel organic. Remember you know your body best, just as you know your children best. When we step onto the mat and let our body move us, we can tap into our intuition in a profound way.

Constructive Rest
Tadasana/Samasthiti (Mountain Pose/Even-Standing
    Pose)
Bitalasana/Marjaryasana (Cat/Cow)
Vrksasana (Tree Pose)
Utkatasana (Chair Pose)
Virabhadrasana II (Warrior II)
Garudasana (Eagle Pose)
Sukhasana with *Sama Vritti Pranayama*
    (Comfortable Cross-Legged Seat)
Upavistha Konasana (Wide-Angle Seated Forward Bend)
Savasana (Corpse Pose)

Reflection

There are a lot of people, parents especially, moving about in this world blissfully unaware, and if not blissful, then silently suffering. I know because I was one of those people for a very long time. I masked my discontent with drinking or drugs or food obsessions. I even masked it with excessive yoga asana, but no matter how many *Chaturangas* you do, things still change, and you realize at a certain point that you have to flow with those changes lest you find yourself fighting an uphill battle and exhausted and miserable every single day.

Life is beautiful, but it is not easy. Parenting is beautiful, but it may well be one of the hardest jobs in the world. It is a mixed bag of highs and lows and ups and downs. Some days feel like an entire year. Other years feel like a day. But when we remain aware—aware of our motivations, aware of external influences, and aware of what our children are going through in that particular moment in time—it may be a little easier to not be swept up by the currents and washed out to sea every time there's some kind of upheaval and turmoil. It is the continual commitment to awareness that can help bring you back to your family, yourself, and your truth when you feel far away.

Yoga reminds us of the hard reality that everything is temporary and everything changes. It reminds us that no matter how much we love our children, they are not ours and they will not be with us forever. Some are only with us a few weeks in the womb, others only a few precious years, and others we are blessed to know our entire lives. But at some point, one of us must go.

And because we have chosen this householder life, this life of being a part of the world and not in some cave somewhere, we have chosen to participate in those vicissitudes every single second of every single day. You are reminded of it every morning that your children wake up as an entirely different person than who they were when they went to sleep. You see it when you roll out your mat and have an entirely different practice than you did the day before, though you may be doing the exact same poses.

It can be overwhelming at first to recognize just how much change there is around us. My anxious side often wants to dig my fingernails into my couch and dig my heels into the floor as if I could stop time. Other times, it wants to rev the gas pedal and catapult forward to the next phase, like when you're reading a book and tempted to jump to the very end. (You didn't do that this time, though, right?)

Yoga offers us an anchor. It reminds us of the truth that despite all the changes happening in the world around us, there is a part of each of us that is ever-present. A part that is always perfect and always whole. This light inside of us, as it is often exemplified, is the same light in our children, and the same light that ignites the sky every morning. It is the light that sparks a new plant budding and encourages the birds to start singing.

It is the light that connects us all together, so that no matter what happens to us in corporeal form, no matter how short a time we may get to be together in this lifetime, we always are, and always will be, connected and a part of one another.

And perhaps by remembering the temporality of it all, we can learn to appreciate even the most challenging of periods. Of course, not in the moment. In the moment, you should cry and yell and grieve and embrace what the mindfulness expert Jon Kabat-Zinn calls "The Full Catastrophe Living" that is parenting. But perhaps a way to come back together more quickly or to reframe even the ugliest of times is the reminder that this is just one blip in the full beautiful picture of our lives and our children's lives.

When I set out to interview all the amazing parents I did, I had no idea the paths I would be taken on or the realizations I would have about my own parenting journey. I knew I was going to talk to people about their day-to-day experiences as parents, but what I quickly realized is that it is actually the totality of all of our lives—from our own childhood to our yoga origin stories, to the cultures we were raised in, to the generation we were born into, to what brought us to raise children in the first place—that helps us become the parents who we are today.

And although everyone is unique and has entirely different approaches and is raising very different children (even within the same family), there is a common thread that helps us weave each of our parenting journeys together, no matter how disparate: it is the choice to live with awareness and seek connection.

Every single parent I speak with, from random people at the park to grandparents to people I meet in the grocery store, all give the exact same advice. We may not vote the same way or have the same viewpoints on certain things, but every single parent I have ever met acknowledges this one indelible truth of parenthood: it all goes by in an instant.

It may not feel like it at the moment when you are having it out with your teenager who yells "I hate you" and storms upstairs. Or when it's two in the morning and you haven't slept for six months with a fussy baby. Or when you must leave an important presentation at work because your little one is sick at school. Yet then it seems so obvious in those most joyful moments, like when you are watching a movie in bed together as a family. Or when you are at your eldest's wedding and having your parent-child dance. Those are the moments we try to hold on to with all of our might while the others we hope to fast-forward.

Can we be present through it all? We have no idea what is coming around the corner in the next moment, let alone day. The only certainty we have is this very moment. And the blessing of a yoga practice (from asana to meditation, to mantra and prayer) is that these are the tools that can bring us back to the moment at any time we choose.

Awareness is like a time machine. It can bring us back to earlier days through choosing certain memories or catapult us to future days through our imagination or it can slow time down and bury us in this very moment. Because if there is any certainty in this world, it is that this moment, just like that beautiful child before you, is fleeting.

ACKNOWLEDGMENTS

This was one of the harder sections to write. There are just so many people I am thankful for, and I am sure I'm going to miss someone. First, I just want to say that I am constantly learning from every single parent I come into contact with, from my fellow moms in Mommy Group to the parents in my neighborhood to random parents at the playground. But of course, the people who have taught me the most, the people who made me a mama, are my sons Jonah and Jacob. I am so grateful that their souls chose these bodies and our family.

Thank you to my husband, Ben, for your unending support. Thank you for listening to me read working chapters out loud on our road trips and never being afraid to give me honest feedback. You are a mirror for me, and I learn so much about myself through you. You make me want to grow and do better because you are so kind and honest. I love sharing this path with you. You are my everything.

Enormous thanks to Kat Rebar (née Heagberg). You know when people say, "I couldn't have done this without you?" Well, I literally couldn't have done this without Kat. She worked tirelessly with me in the beginning to get my book proposal together and was incredibly generous in making the necessary introductions to get this book published. She embodies what it means to support one another.

Jennifer Pastiloff has been a silent player in my career and life since 2008. The universe put us together when we were both leaving jobs we had long defined ourselves by to embark on this path of teaching yoga. Neither of us knew at the time that taking a teacher training and teaching in sweaty gyms would lead us to our true purposes. Seeing Jen blaze forward on her path has always been a guiding light for me and I'm so grateful for her friendship and support.

I think it's kind of amazing that Melanie Salvatore-August and I have still never met in person, though we live one hour away and she has become one of my dearest friends. I truly believe this book wouldn't have happened if she hadn't said a few magical words to me. I watch her as a successful author, mother of three, and devoted yogi, embracing the mess and laughing through the challenges, and I get a clear picture of what is possible.

Beth Frankl, you were able to articulate my vision in a way I never could! Everything I dreamed this book would be, you intuitively knew it should be. I am so grateful for your patience with my many, many emails and your willingness to always educate me about the publishing process. It was truly kismet that we got to work on this together and I am so grateful!

Sarah Stanton, you made a little girl's dreams come true— you made me an author. My entire life, I have wanted to write a book. Thank you for believing in me and this project!

I have had so many incredible yoga teachers over the years. Though I have not taken classes or trainings with some in many, many years (and one is no longer with us), their voices are forever inside of me, guiding me both on my mat and off of it. Thank you especially to Annie Carpenter, Maty Ezraty, Lisa Walford, Joan Hyman, Jeanne Heileman, Ally Hamilton, Sonya Cottle, Bryan Kest, Rudy Mettia, and Anaswara. Not to mention all of my wise colleagues and fellow teachers who I learn from every day just through our friendships.

I can't write a parenting book without thanking my own parents. My father's unending support for me is the invisible hand that has propelled me forward in every area I've ever explored. He is my greatest champion, and I am always amazed that though he is surrounded by the world's most impressive artists and creators, he will always stop to read something I've written. I miss my mom every day and I wish she could have read this book, but it felt as though she was next to me throughout a lot of this and I am so blessed to see her in my sons.

Thank you to my siblings, Josh Ezrin and Geoff Repo, who are some of the best dads I know and whom I learn from every day. A very special thanks to my sister, Jennifer Repo, who another well-known author told me was the best editor she had ever worked with, and I can now confirm. Jenn is never afraid to tell me the truth in life or about my work, and in doing so, it helps me take ownership and grow.

To all of the parents I spoke with for this book: Wow. I can't emphasize enough what a learning experience this was for me. I mean, I knew I'd gather some tidbits, but I didn't think my entire parenting journey would be rerouted in some ways and then reinforced in others. Huge, huge, huge thanks to Paul Teodo, Matthew Sanford, Susan Bordon, Bryan Kest, Anusha

Wijeyakumar, Karly Treacy, MaryBeth LaRue, Jane Austin, Leah Kim, Olivia Barry, Darren Main, Nishanth Selvalingam, Janna Barkin, Dianne Bondy, Erika Trice, David Lynch, Janice Hill, Dawn Stillo, Birgitte Kristen, Nikki Estrada, Kathryn Templeton, Briohny Smyth, Vytas Baskauskus, Jacki Carr, Tamika Caston-Miller, Sara Hess, and Sean Gray.

Many of these parents are experts in their fields and searchable on the web and social media. I encourage you to Google their names and dive deeper into each of their offerings.

And to all the parents I didn't speak directly with but who hugely influence my teachings and support me along this wild path, thank you. Thank you to all of my besties from high school, who modeled for me the type of parent I want to be. Thank you to all of the amazing women from my Kinspace Mommy Group, who have been with me since our babes were little smooshes. And to my new mom friends who though I may have only known a short time, our friendships already run deep.

Last, I want to thank anyone that has ever read my words and said "You should write a book." I doubt myself a lot of the time, and I get in fear around big goals. Every single one of you who has ever said those words to me helped make this happen. I felt you with me at five in the morning each day, cheering me on from the ether, and I thank you all for believing in me and my words. I love writing because it is a way for me to share my most vulnerable spaces, but I especially love it when others recognize themselves and feel seen in that vulnerability. So, thank you.

BIBLIOGRAPHY

INTRODUCTION

Clarke-Fields, Hunter. *Raising Good Humans: A Mindful Guide to Breaking the Cycle of Reactive Parenting and Raising Kind, Confident, Kinds.* Oakland, CA: New Harbinger Publications, 2019.

Roche, Lorin. *The Radiance Sutras: 112 Gateways to the Yoga of Wonder and Delight.* Boulder, CO: Sounds True, 2014.

CHAPTER 1: TO RAISE A LIFE, YOU NEED LIFE-FORCE ENERGY

Druckerman, Pamela. *Bringing Up Bébé: One American Mother Discovers the Wisdom of French Parenting.* New York: Penguin Books, 2014.

Koch, Liz. *The Psoas Book.* Felton, CA: Guinea Pig Publications, 2012.

Sanford, Matthew. *Waking: A Memoir of Trauma and Transcendence.* Emmaus, PA: Rodale Publishing, 2006.

Tham, Elaine, Nora Schneider, and Birit Broekman. "Infant Sleep and Its Relation with Cognition and Growth: A

Narrative Review." *Nature and Science of Sleep* 9 (2017): 135–149. https://doi.org/10.2147/nss.s125992.

Zaccaro, Andrea, Andrea Piarulli, Marco Laurino, Erika Garbella, Danilo Menicucci, Bruno Neri, and Angelo Gemignani. "How Breath-Control Can Change Your Life: A Systematic Review on Psycho-Physiological Correlates of Slow Breathing." *Frontiers in Human Neuroscience* 12 (2018): 353. https://doi.org/10.3389/fnhum.2018.00353.

CHAPTER 2: THE GREATEST GIFT WE CAN GIVE OUR CHILDREN

Augenstein, Tobias, Anna Schneider, Markus Wehler, and Matthias Weigl. "Multitasking Behaviors and Provider Outcomes in Emergency Department Physicians: Two Consecutive, Observational and Multi-Source Studies." *Scandinavian Journal of Trauma, Resuscitation and Emergency Medicine* 29, no. 14 (2021). https://www.doi.org/10.1186/s13049-020-00824-8.

Chandra, Subhash. "Ashram System in Ancient India." University of Delhi, Department of Sanskrit. Accessed August 25, 2021. https://pdfslide.net/documents/ashram-system-in-ancient-documentse-department-of-sanskrit-university-of-delhi.html?page=1.

Hirsch, Patricia, Iring Koch, and Julia Karbach. "Putting a Stereotype to the Test: The Case of Gender Differences in Multitasking Costs in Task-Switching and Dual-Task Situations." *PLoS One* 14, no. 8 (2019). https://doi: 10.1371/journal.pone.0220150.

Roche, Lorin. *Radiance Sutras: 112 Gateways to the Yoga of Wonder and Delight.* Boulder, CO: Sounds True, 2014.

Worringer, Britta, Robert Langner, Iring Koch, Simon Eickhoff, Claudia Eickhoff, and Ferdinand Binkofski. "Common and Distinct Neural Correlates of Dual-Tasking and Task-Switching: A Meta-Analytic Review and a Neuro-Cognitive Processing Model of Human Multitasking." *Brain Structure & Function* 224, no. 5 (2019): 1845–65 https:// doi: 10.1007/s00429-019-01870-4.

Zhang Yue. "Quality Matters More Than Quantity: Parent-Child Communication and Adolescents' Academic Performance." *Frontiers in Psychology* 11, no. 1203 (2020). https:// doi: 10.3389/fpsyg.2020.01203.

CHAPTER 3: HOW TO CHANGE
A PARENT'S MIND

Collardeau, Fanie, Bryony Corbyn, John Abramowitz, Patricia A. Janssen, Sheila Woody, and Nichole Fairbrother. "Maternal Unwanted and Intrusive Thoughts of Infant-Related Harm, Obsessive-Compulsive Disorder and Depression in the Perinatal Period: Study Protocol." *BMC Psychiatry* 19, no. 1 (2019): 94, https://doi.org/10.1186 /s12888-019-2067-x.

Iyengar, B. K. S. *Light on Life: The Yoga Journey to Wholeness, Inner Peace, and Ultimate Freedom.* Emmaus, PA: Rodale, 2006.

Lawrence, Peter, Michelle Craske, Claire Kempton, Anne Stewart, and Alan Stein. "Intrusive Thoughts and Images of Intentional Harm to Infants in the Context of Maternal Postnatal Depression, Anxiety, and OCD." *British Journal of General Practice* 67, no. 661 (2017): 376–77. https://doi .org/10.3399/bjgp17x692105.

Lemay, Virginia, John Hoolahan, and Ashley Buchanan. "Impact of a Yoga and Meditation Intervention on Students' Stress and Anxiety Levels." *American Journal of Pharmaceutical Education* 83, no. 5 (2019): 7001. https://doi.org/10.5688/ajpe7001.

Siegel, Daniel J., and Mary Hartzell. *Parenting from the Inside Out: How a Deeper Self-Understanding Can Help You Raise Children Who Thrive*. Brunswick, Victoria: Scribe Publications, 2018.

Tseng, Julie, and Jordan Poppenk. "Brain Meta-State Transitions Demarcate Thoughts Across Task Contexts Exposing the Mental Noise of Trait Neuroticism." *Nature Communications* 11, 3480 (2020). https://doi.org/10.1038/s41467-020-17255-9.

CHAPTER 4: FINDING CALM
AMID THE CHAOS

Alshak, Mark, and Joe Das. "Neuroanatomy, Sympathetic Nervous System." In StatPearls [Internet]. Treasure Island, FL: StatPearls Publishing, 2021. https://www.ncbi.nlm.nih.gov/books/NBK5421952.

Markham, Laura. *Peaceful Parent, Happy Kid: How to Stop Yelling and Start Connecting*. New York: Perigee, 2012.

Roelofs, Karin. "Freeze for Action: Neurobiological Mechanisms in Animal and Human Freezing." Philosophical Transactions of the Royal Society B: Biological Sciences 372, no. 1718 (2017). https://www.ncbi.nlm.nih.gov/pmc/articles/PMC5332864/.

Siegel, Daniel J., and Mary Hartzell. *Parenting from the Inside Out: How a Deeper Self-Understanding Can Help You Raise*

Children Who Thrive. Brunswick, Victoria: Scribe Publications, 2018.

CHAPTER 5: WHEN CHALLENGES BECOME GIFTS

Academy of Natural Sciences of Drexel University "Butterfly Life Cycle." Accessed August 25, 2021. https://ansp.org /exhibits/onlineexhibits/butterflies/lifecycle/.

Duckworth, Angela. *Grit: The Power of Passion and Perseverance*. New York: Scribner, 2016.

Feurstein, Georg. *The Deeper Dimension of Practice: Theory and Practice*. Boston: Shambhala, 2003.

Iyengar, B. K. S. *Light on the Yoga Sutras of Patanjali*. London: Harper-Collins, 1993.

Julian, Kate. "What Happened to American Childhood?" *The Atlantic*, April 27, 2020,https://www.theatlantic.com/magazine /archive/2020/05/childhood-in-an-anxious-age/609079/.

Satchidananda, Sri Swami. *The Yoga Sutras of Patanjali: Translation and Commentary*. Buckingham, VA: Integral Yoga Publications, 1978.

CHAPTER 6: SETTING LIMITS WITH LOVE

Alia-Klein, Nelly, Rita Z. Goldstein , Dardo Tomasi, Lei Zhang, Stephanie Fagin-Jones, Frank Telang, Gene-Jack Wang, Joanna S. Fowler, and Nora D. Volkow. "What Is in a Word? No versus Yes Differentially Engage the Lateral Orbitofrontal Cortex." *Emotion* 7, no. 3 (2007): 649-59. https:// doi:10.1037/1528-3542.7.3.649.

Lamott, Anne. *Operating Instructions: A Journal of My Son's First Year*. New York: Anchor Books, 2005.

Sanvictores, Terrence, and Magda D. Mendez, "Types of Parenting Styles and Effects on Children." In StatPearls [Internet]. Treasure Island, FL: StatPearls Publishing, 2022. https://www.ncbi.nlm.nih.gov/books/NBK568743/.

Siegel, Daniel J., and Mary Hartzell. *Parenting from the Inside Out: How a Deeper Self-Understanding Can Help You Raise Children Who Thrive*. Brunswick, Victoria: Scribe Publications, 2018.

Tsabary, Shefali. *The Conscious Parent: Transforming Ourselves, Empowering our Children*. Vancouver, BC: Namaste Publishing, 2010.

CHAPTER 7: IF YOU LOVE SOMETHING, LET IT GO

Carrera, Jaganath. *Inside the Yoga Sutras*. New York: Northpoint Press, 2006.

Doucleff, Michaeleen. *Hunt, Gather, Parent: What Ancient Cultures Can Teach Us About the Lost Art of Raising Happy, Helpful Little Humans*. New York: Avid Reader Press, 2021.

Gerber, Magda. *Your Self-Confident Baby: How to Encourage Your Child's Natural Abilities from the Very Start*. New York: John Wiley & Sons, 1976.

Katie, Byron. *Loving What Is: Four Questions That Will Change Your Life*. New York: Harmony Books, 2002.

Tigunait, Pandit Rajmani. *The Secret of the Yoga Sutras: Samadhi Pada*. Honesdale, PA: Himalayan Institute, 2014.

Warner, Michelle Marie. "How to Detach with Love in Your Relationships." *PS I Love You* (blog), April 23, 2020, https://psiloveyou.xyz/how-to-detach-with-love-in-your-relationships-324fc8684de0.

CHAPTER 8: LIVING IN HARMONY

Chaudhary, Anand, and Neetu Singh. "Contribution of World Health Organization in the Global Acceptance of Ayurveda." *Journal of Ayurveda and Integrative Medicine* 2, no. 4 (2011): 179. https://doi.org/10.4103/0975-9476.90769

Patwardhan, Bhushan. "The Quest for Evidence-Based Ayurveda: Lessons Learned." *Current Science* 102, no. 10 (2012): 1406–17. http://www.jstor.org/stable/24107798.

Saini, Anu. "Physicians of Colonial India (1757–1900)." *Journal of Family Medicine and Primary Care* 5, no. 3 (2016): 528. https://doi.org/10.4103/2249-4863.197257.

Silcox, Katie. *Healthy Happy Sexy: Ayurveda Wisdom for Modern Women.* New York: Atria Paperback, 2015.

CHAPTER 9: THE SHARENTING DILEMMA

Cornwall, Gail. "Perfectionism Can Become a Vicious Cycle in Families Mothers and Fathers Risk Passing Down This Tendency to The Next Generation, Creating a Pattern of Dissatisfaction." *The Atlantic*, July 19, 2021, https://www.theatlantic.com/family/archive/2021/07/family-other-oriented-perfectionism-parents-child/619461/.

"Social Media Use in 2021." Pew Research Center, April 7, 2021, https://www.pewresearch.org/internet/2021/04/07/social-media-use-in-2021/.

Riehm, Kira E., Kenneth A. Feder, Kayla N. Tormohlen, Rosa M. Crum, Andrea S. Young, Kerry M. Green, Lauren R. Pacek, Lareina N. La Flair, and Ramin Mojtabai. "Associations Between Time Spent Using Social Media and Internalizing and Externalizing Problems among US Youth."

JAMA Psychiatry, 76, no. 12: 1266–73 (2019). doi:10.1001/jamapsychiatry.2019.2325.

Viner, Russell M., Aswathikutty Gireesh, Neza Stiglic, Lee D. Hudson, Anne-Lise Goddings, Joseph L. Ward, and Dasha E. Nicholls. "Roles of Cyberbullying, Sleep, and Physical Activity in Mediating the Effects of Social Media Use on Mental Health and Wellbeing Among Young People in England: A Secondary Analysis of Longitudinal Data." *The Lancet. Child & Adolescent Health* 3, no. 10 (2019): 685–96. https://doi.org/10.1016/S2352-4642(19)30186-5.

CHAPTER 10: THE END IS ALSO THE BEGINNING

Badal, Kelly Phillips. "In Photos: A Gorgeous Indian City That Welcomes the Dead and Dying." *Travel & Leisure*, December 8, 2015, https://www.travelandleisure.com/trip-ideas/adventure-travel/varanasi-india-death-celebrations.

Constable, Pamela. "The Mystery of the Hundreds of Bodies Found in India's Ganges River." *The Washington Post*, May 22, 2010. https://www.washingtonpost.com/world/asia_pacific/india-coronavirus-ganges-river-bodies/2021/05/21/73cbced6-b811-11eb-bc4a-62849cf6cca9_story.html.

Iyengar, B. K. S. *Light on Life: The Yoga Journey to Wholeness, Inner Peace, and Ultimate Freedom*. Emmaus, PA: Rodale Press, 2006.

McBride, Pete. "The Pyres of Varanasi: Breaking the Cycle of Death and Rebirth." *National Geographic*, August 7, 2014, https://www.nationalgeographic.com/photography/article/the-pyres-of-varanasi-breaking-the-cycle-of-death-and-rebirth.

RESOURCES

Please note that neither the author nor Shambhala Publications have affiliations with any of the below companies, brands, books, or resources. They are simply offerings for you to dive deeper into the discussed subjects if you choose.

INTRODUCTION
Sanskrit Pronunciation Guides

FPMT Translation Services: A Guide to Sanskrit Transliteration and Pronunciation, https://fpmt.org/wp-content/uploads/education/translation/guide_to_sanskrit_transliteration_and_pronunciation.pdf

CHAPTER 1: TO RAISE A LIFE, YOU NEED LIFE-FORCE ENERGY

Mind Body Solutions, https://www.mindbodysolutions.org/

CHAPTER 3: HOW TO CHANGE A PARENT'S MIND
Foster Care and Adoption Resources

Extraordinary Families: Foster Care & Adoption, https://www.extraordinaryfamilies.org

National Foster Parent Association, https://nfpaonline.org
/FPResources

CHAPTER 4
FINDING CALM AMID THE CHAOS
Postpartum Mental Health Resources

Postpartum Support International, https://www.postpartum
.net

Substance Abuse and Mental Health Services Administration
(SAMHSA), https://www.samhsa.gov

Nervous System Charts and Resources

Mentone Educational: Anatomical Models and Education Sup-
plies, https://www.mentone-educational.com.au/charts
-and-posters/anatomical-charts/the-nervous-system-chart

Merck Manual, Overview of the Autonomic Nervous System,
https://www.merckmanuals.com/home/brain,-spinal
-cord,-and-nerve-disorders/autonomic-nervous-system
-disorders/overview-of-the-autonomic-nervous-system

CHAPTER 5: WHEN CHALLENGES
BECOME GIFTS
LGBTQ Children Online Support Organizations

Gender Spectrum Organization, https://genderspectrum.org
The Trevor Project, https://www.thetrevorproject.org/explore/

Additional Reading

Brill, Stephanie, and Rachel Pepper. *The Transgender Child:
A Handbook for Families and Professionals.* Hoboken, NJ:
Cleis Press, 2022.

Ehrensaft, Diane. *Gender Born, Gender Made: Raising Healthy Gender-Noncomforming Children*. New York: Experiment LLC, 2011.

———. *The Gender Creative Child: Pathways for Nurturing and Supporting Children Who Live Outside Gender Boxes*. New York: Experiment LLC, 2016.

Pessin-Whedbee, Brook. *Who Are You?: The Kids Guide to Gender Identity*. London: Jessica Kingsley, 2016.

CHAPTER 7: IF YOU LOVE SOMETHING, LET IT GO

RIE Resources

Janet Lansbury Podcast: Unruffled, https://www.janetlansbury.com/tag/podcasts/

Resources for Infant Educarers® (RIE®), https://www.rie.org

CHAPTER 9: THE SHARENTING DILEMMA

Kathryn Templeton's "Simple Self-Care Tips for Parents"

Kathryn Templeton has created for this book an easy way for you to get started (or restarted) with a sustainable daily routine that is both cleansing and nurturing.

Choosing to begin each day with self-care keeps your three tanks full (nourishment, sleep, and judicious use of energy) and will help you navigate life's stressors with more steadiness and grace.

Begin with just one or two items at first when building your daily routine. From there, you can add on every few days or even weeks. The order below is simply a guideline, based on feedback from other busy parents like you. Feel free to do these in any order that works for you!

1. **Wake before the sun rises:** When you rise with the sun, you'll likely find you feel lighter and more energetic than if you wake post sunrise. Don't believe us? Try it for a week and see.

2. **Say a prayer or positive affirmation (see chapter 3) before leaving your bed:** Bring your mind into the day from a place of gratitude and intention.

3. **Scrape your tongue:** In Ayurveda, *ama* refers to the "toxins" or "goo" that can build up, and according to Ayurveda, can lead to potential health problems down the road, not to mention bad breath. Scraping the tongue removes this debris and is said to stimulate digestion.

4. **Neti pot with neti salt:** This is intended to cleanse the nose, throat, and mouth of congestion. Clearing congestion will help you both breathe and think with greater ease.

5. **Oil pulling:** This is intended to support gum health and decrease inflammation. Warm a tablespoon of pure unrefined, organic sesame oil (you can mix in a tablespoon of water if desired) and using your clean index finger, dab some on your gums and gently massage. Swish the remainder in your mouth for as long as you can, up to twenty minutes. Sarah likes to do this when showering. Spit the excess into the toilet to prevent clogged drains.

6. **Drink water:** Before having any other liquid or food, drink a glass of room temperature water. To aid in evacuation, try a cup of hot water with lemon (or lime, if you naturally run hot) and raw honey.

7. **Dry brushing:** This not only helps us have glowing skin but it is also said to awaken the mind and help with lymph drainage. Use a dry washcloth if you don't have a brush. Take your dry brush (preferably a vegetable bristle) and stroke long on the long bones and in a circle on the joints, with small round strokes on your tummy and chest. Some Ayurvedic practitioners believe that brushing in the direction of the heart helps support the lymphatic system.

8. **Abhyanga (oil massage) and bathing:** This may feel like the most luxurious of all of our suggestions and that's okay because you deserve it! Have oil warming in the sink while you're dry brushing. Many people use coconut or sesame oil. Next, smooth the oil on your skin using the same process you used for dry brushing. You can oil the tops of your feet, but avoid rubbing your soles (no parents slipping in the shower, please!). Afterward, hop in the shower or take a bath. The oil tends to stick to your skin, so consider using an old towel and dressing in dark clothes that you're okay with getting a little stained.

9. **Food sadhana:** Remember *sadhana* means "practice," so please don't worry if you can only do one or two of these. Ayurveda believes food is our medicine. A lot of these suggestions are review from chapter 9, but we consolidated them here for easy reference:

   - Before you eat, give thanks.
   - Eat warm and moist foods.
   - Have your heaviest meal at lunchtime.
   - Choose seasonal foods when possible.

- Cook fresh foods when you're able instead of reheating frozen or premade foods.
- Eat somewhere calm. (It may be best to eat before everyone else is up!)
- Chew mindfully.

Ayurvedic Practitioners
Offering Online Consultations

Dr. Shiva Mohan, Ayurveda by Siva
https://members.ayurvedabysiva.com

Dr. Vaidya Jayagopal Parla (Dr. Jay), Athreya Ayurveda
https://www.athreyaayurveda.com/

Mela Gaskins Butcher, Center for Ayurveda
http://centerforayurveda.com

Online Ayurveda Courses

The School of Yoga: Yoga and Ayurveda Workshop led by Jeanne Heileman and Joan Hyman, https://www.schoolof.yoga
Ayurveda 101 on Yoga International, https://yogainternational .com/ecourse/player/ayurveda-101

Additional Reading

Egidio, Rhonda. *365 Days of Ayurveda for Lifelong Radiant Health: Daily Wisdom & Simple Tips for Physical, Emotional & Spiritual Well-Being.* Radiant Life Press, 2020.
Mohan, Shiva. *Ayurveda for Yoga Teachers & Students: Bringing Ayurveda into Your Life and Practice.* London: Singing Dragon, 2019.

Yarema, Thomas, Daniel Rhoda, and Chef Johnny Brannigan. *Eat-Taste-Heal: An Ayurvedic Cookbook for Modern Living.* Kapaa, HI: Five Elements Press, 2006.

Additional Dosha Quizzes

Banyan Botanicals, https://www.banyanbotanicals.com/info/dosha-quiz/

Yoga International, https://yogainternational.com/article/view/dosha-quiz

Chopra Center Quiz, https://chopra.com/dosha-quiz

CHAPTER 10: THE END IS ALSO THE BEGINNING

National Alliance of Mental Illness, "How to Have a Healthy Relationship with Social Media." https://www.nami.org/Blogs/NAMI-Blog/February-2019/How-to-Have-a-Healthy-Relationship-with-Social-Media

Healthline.com, "What Is Social Media Addiction?" https://www.healthline.com/health/social-media-addiction

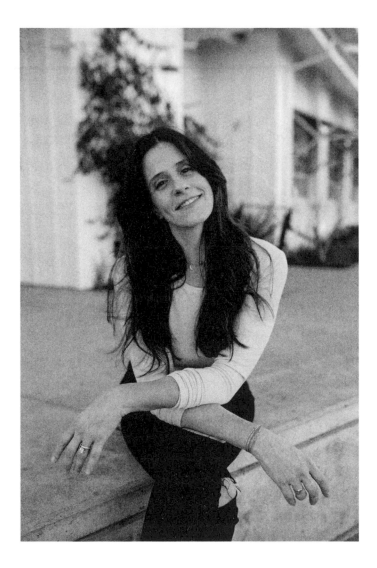

ABOUT THE AUTHOR

Sarah Ezrin is an author, world-renowned yoga educator, and content creator based in the San Francisco Bay Area, where she lives with her husband, two sons, and their dog. Her willingness to be unabashedly honest and vulnerable along with her innate wisdom make her writing, classes, and social media great sources of healing and inner peace for many people.

Sarah is a frequent contributor to *Yoga Journal* and *LA Yoga Magazine* as well as for the award-winning media organization Yoga International. She also writes for parenting sites Healthline-Parenthood, Scary Mommy, and Motherly. She has been interviewed for her expertise by the *Wall Street Journal*, *Forbes*, and Bustle.com and has appeared on television on NBC News. Sarah is a highly accredited yoga teacher. A world traveler since birth, she leads teacher trainings, workshops, and retreats locally in her home state of California and across the globe.

Sarah brings a wide spectrum of life experiences into everything she does. She is unafraid of sharing all sides of herself and her life and does so in the hope of giving others permission to be their most authentic selves as well. At this time, when honest self-awareness is so important, Sarah's is an essential and exemplary voice.

For more information on Sarah, please visit her website www.sarahezrinyoga.com. You can also follow her on Instagram @sarahezrinyoga and TikTok @sarahezrin.